AF647674

Psychological Perspectives on Chronic Illnesses

About the Author

Anubhuti Dubey is Associate Professor of the Department of Psychology, D.D.U. Gorakhpur University. Her areas of interest include health psychology, applied social psychology, counseling and women studies. She is on the editorial board of "Indian Journal of Social Science Researches". She had completed the ICSSR research project on "Psychological Dynamics of Health and Illness in Women of Eastern Uttar Pradesh". She had received gold medals at undergraduate and post-graduate levels. She is a Master Trainer for Training HIV/AIDS counselors under GFATM-Round 7.

Psychological Perspectives on Chronic Illnesses

Dr. (Mrs.) Anubhuti Dubey,
Reader,
Department of Psychology,
D.D.U. Gorakhpur University,
Gorakhpur

Concept Publishing Company Pvt. Ltd.
New Delhi-110059

© Dr. (Mrs.) Anubhuti Dubey

All rights reserved. No part of this work may be reproduced, stored, adapted, or transmitted in any form or by any means, electronic, mechanical, photocopying, micro-filming recording or otherwise, or translated in any language, without the prior written permission of the copyright owner and the publisher. The book is sold subject to the condition that it shall not, by way of trade or otherwise, be lent, resold, hired out, or otherwise circulated without the prior publisher's written consent in any form of binding or cover other than that in which it is published.

The views and opinions expressed in this book are author(s) own and the facts reported by him/her have been verified to the extent possible, and the publishers are not in any way liable for the same.

ISBN-13 : 978-81-8069-842-2

First Published 2012

Published and Printed by

Concept Since 1974

Concept Publishing Company Pvt. Ltd.
A/15-16, Commercial Block, Mohan Garden
New Delhi-110059 (India)
T: 25351460, 25351794, *F*: 091-11-25357109
E: publishing@conceptpub.com, W: www.conceptpub.com
Editorial Office: H-13, Bali Nagar, New Delhi-110 015, India.

Cataloging in Publication Data--*Courtesy:* D.K. Agencies (P) Ltd. <docinfo@dkagencies.com>

Dubey, Anubhuti.
Psychological perspectives on chronic illnesses / Anubhuti Dubey.
p. cm.
Originally presented as the author's thesis (Ph. D.)—Deen Dayal Upadhyay Gorakhpur University.
Includes bibliographical references (p.) and index.
ISBN 9788180698422

1. Chronic diseases—India—Gorakhpur—Psychological aspects. 2. Chronic diseases—Patients—India—Gorakhpur—Psychology. I. Title.

DDC 616.009542 23

Dedicated

to

My beloved

Parents

Foreword

Health psychology is amongst the most important developments in the later part of 20th century (Taylor, 1995). It has retained its prominent status in the 21st century, because man has conquered many acute illnesses and infectious diseases in the last century. The diseases which overwhelm people, cut the life short, or change the course of their lives, are mostly those diseases which have their roots in lifestyle. Managing them requires lifestyle changes, hence, there is need to study and do research in health psychology.

Perhaps in the ancient times man believed in the unity of body and mind, but with the advances in sciences, bodily factors came to be considered as most relevant in explaining the cause of illness and its treatment. This duality between mind and body became the basis of medical progress. This view continued roughly for 300 years in western medical science. The ancient Indian view—Ayurveda defined health as a state of delight—spiritual, physical and mental well-being. Nevertheless, the impact of western bio-medical philosophy was so pervasive and powerful that Ayurveda had been put on the back shelf and along with it the holistic thinking was also overlooked.

Freud (1856-1939) drew attention to the unconscious conflicts which caused many symptoms of diseases, like conversion hysteria. Later the concept of psychosomatic diseases was developed, physiological mechanisms were postulated to provide linkage between conflict and disorder. This movement was criticized on the basis of many grounds but it did bring to focus the relation between body and mind. All the above-mentioned factors brought about acceptance of Health psychology.

Health psychology had become an upcoming field in India also, but it was still amongst the developing fields when

Dr. Anubhuti Dubey (nee Pandey) joined the movement. Theoretical development was in nascent stage, hence which psychosocial variables should be studied was not clear. Indigenous tools were not readily available and dealing with people who were already upset and perturbed with their illness was not the least of the problems.

This book is the fruit of the young tree. The sapling was planted when Dr. Anubhuti Dubey was a master's student in the department of psychology. Based on her first research paper on the role of some psychological variables on coping with chronic disease, she was fascinated with the idea that a diverse array of health protective and disease preventive factors were embedded in the social and behavioural milieu of people and not caused by bodily dysfunction or infections alone. She worked towards her Ph.D. under my guidance on the "Role of Some Psychological Variables in Chronic Illnesses". The present book is based on that work. She designed her investigation based on psychosocial model and studied patients suffering from cancer, diabetes, and coronary heart disease. Tools employed are by and large, indigenous and are, therefore, suited to the population under study.

Earlier studies had indicated that some psychological variables like optimism, showed varied influences on behaviour, depending upon the culture of the people under study. On the other hand, other variables like future orientation had rarely been studied in the context of health psychology. Dr. Anubhuti Dubey investigated the impact of such variables on people fighting with deadly diseases. Her findings will now be available to a wider audience and may help in putting smiles back on the faces of some sufferers. Psychologists, health workers, health counsellors and researchers in social sciences will find the book beneficial and useful.

43A Jail Road
Gita Garden
Gorakhpur

Dr. (Mrs.) Adesh Agarwal
Formerly: Professor and Head
Department of Psychology and
Dean Faculty of Arts
D.D.U. Gorakhpur University
Gorakhpur

Acknowledgements

I am privileged to have conducted my Ph.D. thesis work under the supervision of Prof. (Mrs.) Adesh Agarwal, Head, Department of Psychology, D.D.U. Gorakhpur University. My supervisor, esteemed teacher and a versatile genius blessed with unique combination of elegance and eloquence. This entire work is due to her sincere suggestions, creative criticism and innovative ideas. Her scientific approach and scholarly guidance was responsible for steady progress of my project. Her motherly advice has always produced appreciations and rewards for me. Each and every word spoken by her to me has always enlightened me.

I pay my deepest and sincere regards to Prof. R.A. Agarwal, ex-pro-Vice-Chancellor, D.D.U. Gorakhpur University. He always encouraged me to complete my work. He has given me suggestions not for this work only, but for the life as a whole.

I am grateful to **Prof. A.N. Tripathi, Prof. P.S.N. Tiwari, Dr. Rakesh Pandey** and **Mr. Dhananjaya Kumar** for their encouragement and help. All of them have been a constant source of inspiration. I especially express my thanks to Prof. P.S.N. Tiwari for his calm and compassionate attitude, which was like cool and refreshing showers of spring in a mid-summer day. I am especially grateful to Dr. Rakesh Pandey. His unparalleled calibre, experience and knowledge have influenced me in more ways than one.

I express my sincere appreciation and heartfelt gratitude towards my father and mother-in-law, **Sri Daya Shanker Dubey** and **Mrs. Urmila Dubey** for their invaluable support and patience. I could not have completed this work without their support.

Multiple resources are important in health and illness. This work is hoped to give an insight to effective health promotion and maintenance of well being even in the wake of adversity.

Anubhuti Dubey

Preface

The field of Health Psychology is growing steadily and great advances in research have been made, especially using the biopsychosocial model. The psychosocial factors exert both protective and adverse effects on health depending on the nature and intensity of the factor.

The chapter of introduction provides an overview of the concepts of health and illness in western and eastern systems of medicine and psychology. The models of health and the three major chronic diseases namely—cancer, diabetes and heart disease were also discussed. The chapter reviews the researches on the role of psychological characteristics in chronic illness. The coping approaches to overcome stress and maintaining quality of life were outlined.

The method chapter deals with the sample taken for the research work and the details of the measures used with the descriptions of the procedure utilized for the study. In the results chapter the analysis of the empirical finding is being presented. It indicated the association of chronic stressors with psychological characteristics.

In the chapter of discussion the linkages in chronic disease related stress to psychological characteristics and well being were shown. Coping strategies to deal with chronic disease is being illustrated. For the intention and rehabilitation of chronically ill people the findings are very pertinent as it provides the effective coping strategies, enhancement of psychological qualities and being positively maintaining quality of life and leading to satisfaction.

I am short of words to express the immense love and blessings which have been bestowed upon me by my parents, **Dr. V.K. Pandey** and **Mrs. Urmila Pandey.** Their affection and backing were the source of constant encouragement in successful completion of the present work. To them, I bow my head in all veneration.

I am overwhelmed while expressing gratitude to my younger brother **Harsh Bardhan** and my younger sister **Abhiruchi**, for their love, affection and moral support in carrying out this research work.

My gratitude to my husband, **Dr. Ran Vijay Dubey**, Neuro-Surgeon for his moral support. He was always near me in deed and need. I got his love, support and cooperation at all hours.

I owe special thanks to my son **Shubhag Vibhu** for his supportive attitude towards me. So many times I had been harsh to him because of work pressure and curtailed his time which I should have devoted to him, but he always adjusted with all this. His one sweet smile inspired and encouraged me to work again. Thanks Beta.

Last but not the least, I wish to thank all my patients and other participants who as a subjects of my present endeavour gave selfless time and cooperation. Thanks are a poor recompense for all that I have received but I hope it will prove adequate to a generous heart.

Anubhuti Dubey (Pandey)

Contents

List of Tables

Introduction

WHO (1947) had defined health as "a state of complete physical, mental and social well-being and not merely the absence of disease or infirmity." Biologist and Philosopher Rene Dubos (1968) further elaborated the definition of health as given by WHO as "a quality of life, involving social, emotional, spiritual and biological fitness on the part of the individual which results from adaptations to the environment."

The term "Health" now denotes a concept which includes several components, which encompasses many different aspects of life. Historically, health has been considered as the absence of disease and physical fitness. Therefore, the earlier models of health in the western science of medicine have illustrated the physical condition of the body. The Western models of health are as follows—

Biomedical Model

This model states that a normally functioning individual infected by some pathogenic stimulus like, an infection can be treated directly by physical intervention. It further says that cure works with or without the assistance of the patient. Cure is purely physical and is not influenced by the thoughts or emotional state of the patient. This model assumes that disease and their treatment are largely independent of psychological and social processes. The important assumptions of this model are that disordered cells and chemical imbalance cause illness, illness is the consequence of malfunction and other factors may not be responsible for the development of illness, mind and body are two separate entities.

This traditional biomedical model is effective in treating diseases, but one of the major limitations of this model is that it has not incorporated the knowledge that thoughts and emotions can speed up development of disease or promote the cure process. The potential power of thoughts and emotions in the process of disease and health was realized later on. Efforts have, therefore, been made to identify the interactions between psychological and disease related pathophysiological processes.

Biobehavioural Model

This model views that a person's psychological processes like his thoughts, emotions and spoken words, interact with cultural and social environment, allow informational changes and it has an impact on outcomes. Although, in this model the interactions among the treatment, pathogen and host and the social environment and psychosocial functioning, as process that affect treatment outcome, have been emphasized, but still treatment acts to alter the disease state only.

Biopsychosocial Model

This model of health and illness assumes that in the maintenance of health and treatment of illness, the biological, psychological and social factors are all equally important (Engel, 1977, 1980, Schwartz, 1982). The emphasis of this model is upon the fact that health and illnesses are caused by multiple factors and produce multiple effects. This model maintains that mind and body cannot be distinguished in matters of health and illness because both have apparent effects on a person's health status. This model clearly implies that a practitioner must understand the social and psychological factors that contribute to illness in order to treat it appropriately (Schwartz, 1982). The best feature of this model is that it not only suggests ways of treating illness but also give suggestions about how to maintain a healthy status. The model says that one can understand health habits only in their psychological and social contexts. These contexts may maintain a poor health habit or without appropriate modifications, can facilitate the development of healthy ones. For ill people, this model suggests that biological, psychological and social factors all contribute to recovery and adaptation to chronic illness.

This model has attracted the attention of many psychologists, social scientists and physicians and has led to investigations exposing the relationships in psychosocial variables and health.

Indian View of Health

The Indian medicinal systems like Ayurveda and Yoga emphasized that complete harmony among mind, body and spirit leads to an ideal state of health. Ayurveda states that body is constituted with three basic components: *Vaat* (gases), *Pitta* (acids) and *Kaph* (Phlegm) and most of the health related problems are only due to imbalance amongst these three. In Ayurveda, regularity in daily life activities and proper balanced diet are considered as important as medicine. Ayurveda also realize the powerful impact of emotional state on body and recommends positive thinking as essential for well-being. According to Ayurveda staying healthy is dependent upon biological factors only but equally contingent upon lifestyle, cultural beliefs, health habits, family support and other such factors.

D. Sinha (1990) examined ancient Indian treatise to understand the concept of health in Indian tradition and found that Indian conceptualization of health is broadbased and holistic. He quoted "Sushrut", the ancient proponent of the traditional system of medicine and surgery, who defined health as 'prasannanmeddriyamanah swasthwa' which means health is a state of delight or a feeling spiritual, physical and mental well-being. The essential characteristics of healthy person is possessing in right quantities (sama) of four: *samadosh* (defects or weaknesses), *samaagni* (digestive quality), *samadhatua* (semen) and *malkriya* (normal bodily functions). This conceptualization perceives health in a holistic manner, a total well-being and feeling of happiness. Sankhya philosophy and *Bhagvad Gita* also emphasized the maintenance of balance or equilibrium in all functioning.

Chronic Illnesses

Health related problems are medically categorized into two categories: (i) acute, and (ii) chronic. Acute problems usually begin abruptly, are easily diagnosed, are of short duration and respond to a specific treatment, e.g., cold or chicken pox or viral fever etc.

Chronic illnesses are different. They begin and proceed slowly. The term chronic illness is used to describe a group of health conditions that last a long time. The root word of chronic is "chronos" which refers to time. Chronic illnesses have multiple causes varying over time. Heredity, lifestyle factors, invasive environmental and physiological factors may all contribute in the development of chronic illness. In most of the chronic illness conditions the long term effects may be difficult to predict. This lack of predictive pattern is a major characteristic of most chronic illnesses. Chronic illness challenges every aspect of life. The more serious the illness is, the greater the challenge it imposes.

About half of the Indian population lives with some chronic health condition. The prevalence pattern of chronic illnesses all-over the world is similar, accounting for over 80 per cent deaths worldwide; therefore, large number of people are living, working and coping with illness in their daily life.

The list of chronic diseases includes diabetes, cancer, irritable bowel syndrome, heart diseases, arthritis, inflammatory bowel disease, asthma, epilepsy etc. Chronic illnesses start at cellular level. Though biological causes differ, the symptoms they cause are similar, like fatigue, pain, loss of energy, loss of appetite, sleeplessness, and restlessness etc. These symptoms often interfere with everyday life and may require a change in existing pattern of life. Other common problems with chronic illnesses are depression, anxiety, fear and concern for the future. Physical limitations and decreased work ability can lead to financial difficulties. The important thing is that similarities exist among chronic illnesses as people suffering from different chronic diseases must learn the central management tasks and skills to live and deal effectively with disease. Chronic illnesses have serious impact on persons and their families, as such long-term illnesses lead to abandonment of careers, break-up of marriages, and loss of self-esteem and personal worth. The patients may find their personal ambitions and hopes to be on the edge. These changes have profound psychological impact on the victim as well as on their families. Anxiety, depression, anger, hopelessness, loneliness, and fears can become full-time engagements. These emotions have significant effect on the body and its capacity to cope with illness and to heal. The drastic mood swings become the part of life. People with chronic and multiple physical and emotional problems do better when medication is combined with individual and family psychological support.

Chronic illnesses consist of incurable diseases which can only be managed by the patient himself along with all those around him like, his doctor, family members and peer group. Review of literature indicates a noticeable increase in the prevalence rate of chronic illnesses not only in India, but all-over the world. Till 20th century the chief cause of illness and death was acute or short term medical disorders like, pneumonia, malaria, flu and other viral or bacterial diseases. Although some diseases had longer course like, tuberculosis, but due to modernization, changes in lifestyle and health habits etc., the occurrence rate of chronic illnesses like, diabetes, cancer, cardiovascular diseases, also known as lifestyle diseases, is now very high. Now these diseases have become the main contributor of disability and death. Chronic illnesses are typically dangerous and burdensome for two main reasons—

(i) The person who is diagnosed with any chronic illness has to live rest of his life with the disease and has to manage it on day-to-day basis.

(ii) As the chronic illness develops further it not only damages the affected region but may also cause a number of other complications e.g., in case of diabetes, the diabetic patients generally suffer from complications like, retinopathy, nephropathy or neuropathy, along with insufficient manufacture or improper utilization of insulin.

In the light of these two above-mentioned reasons it can be easily understood that chronic illnesses are those diseases in which social and psychological factors can influence the coping efforts of the patients, the course of disease, and patients' quality of life. Patients may live with chronic disease for many years. Psychological and social issues arise in this connection. Chronic illness affects patient's positive mental state, threatens him to think about his future, induce feeling of hopelessness, and helplessness, severely hamper daily activities and routine, and may shaken overall quality of life. Besides these psychological factors, chronic illnesses also affect the family functioning. So, positive psychological state of patient and degree of social support are important for management of chronic illness over the years.

WHO (2002) in its report estimated that 29 per cent of deaths worldwide (16.7 million deaths) were due to Cardiovascular Diseases (CVD). The prevalence rate of chronic diseases in India is increasing very rapidly, e.g., at present around 50 million Indian population is suffering from blood pressure and other cardiac disorders. During the last 35 years the prevalence rate of Coronary Artery Disease (CAD) has increased from 3.45 per cent to 9.45 per cent in urban areas. Even in the rural areas this has increased to become just double, i.e. from 2 per cent to 4 per cent. There is a projection that by the year 2015, CAD might come out to be as the largest cause of death (Indrayan, 2005). It is also very alarming that about 25 per cent of the total heart patients are around 40 years in age, which means the working population of India (Parasher, 2000) and the heart diseases had the highest prevalence (6.6%) of the total population along with respiratory illnesses in India (Anand, 2000). Heart attack was the third most important cause of death among rural Indian women (Raman Kumar, 2004). The picture of the prevalence rate of diabetes is not much different from CAD in India. Nearly, 20 million people in India are diabetics and their number is likely to reach 52 million by 2025. It is also very damaging that a sufficient number of diabetic patients also suffer from coronary artery heart problems. The prevalence rate of coronary heart disease in diabetics is 20 to 25 per cent and incidence of silent heart attack is 30 to 40 per cent as stated by a heart specialist. According to World Health Organization report, Indians are going to have the highest incidence of CAD in the world *(Times of India, 1999)*. Risk factors arise from determinants and are directly linked to a disease in a causal fashion, although not everyone with the risk factor develops the disease. Risk factors include smoking, high blood pressure, malnutrition, obesity, hyperlipidemia, lack of physical exercise, and beta-hemolytic streptococcal infection. Many of the determinants of CVD are shared with cancer, diabetes, and chronic obstructive disease.

The general course of these chronic illnesses in India includes changing lifestyle, unmindful modernization, obesity etc. But the major risk factor for CHD constituted smoking or tobacco chewing. About 75 per cent of CHD are smokers and tobacco chewers. Tobacco and diabetes are closely linked and diabetic smokers head for all sorts of complications including kidney damage, blindness and strokes *(Times of India, 1999)*. In India it is estimated that presently 19.4 million individuals are affected by diabetes, which is likely to go up to 57.2 million by the year 2025 (Pradeepa, Deepa and Mohan, 2002).

The scenario for cancer is also similar. According to Cancer Society of India every year around 80,000 new cases of cancer are detected in Indian cities. This disease toll around 35,000 lives every year. From 1990 onwards the cancer death rate has increased to 18 per cent. In 1970s in India the prevalence rate of breast cancer was 20 per 1 lakh ladies but now it is 28.6 per 1 lakh, which means there is a 50 per cent increase in this rate. The alarming thing is that in the maximum cases of breast or uterus cancer the average age is between 35 to 45 years. Similarly in males there is an alarming increase in oral cancer *(India Today, 2000)*.

Cancer

The name "Cancer" has been given to a set of more than hundred immunologic faulty functioning diseases characterized by the uncontrolled growth and spread of abnormal cells. The causes of cancer are poorly understood, because a number of factors make the study of cancer very difficult. Researchers and scientists are not very sure why malignant cells spread and dysfunction in DNA occurs. But they have given several propositions for the cellular changes that result in cancer. Some of this are:

(a) Some spontaneous error during cell reproduction may results cancer.
(b) Some external agent or agents that enter a normal cell and initiate the cancerous process, e.g. environmental factors such as radiation, chemicals, hormonal drugs, immune suppressant drugs.
(c) Some cancer causing genes may produce cancer.

Some species are more vulnerable to cancer than others because some cancers are species specific, e.g. monkeys get very few cancers. Many cancers run in families, e.g. colon and breast cancer. Some cancers are ethnically linked, e.g. malignant melanoma in Anglo men in USA. Some cancers are culturally linked through lifestyle, e.g. high rate of breast cancer among American women. Therefore, some of the most suspected causes of cancer, which in combination increases the risk of cancer, are—Viral factors, Medical factors, Biological factors, Chemicals in food, Social and psychological factors, and Occupational/Environmental factors.

The complex interaction of heredity predisposition, lifestyle and environment on the development of cancer makes it very difficult to determine a single cause of cancer. Cancers of the breast, stomach, colon, prostrate, uterus, ovaries, Hodgkin's disease and lungs do appear to run in families. Occupational hazards, like nickel benzene, arsenic and vinyl chloride have been shown to be carcinogens for human being, if it have a continuous and high level of exposure. Similarly, sodium nitrate, a food additive particularly used to preserve and give colour to food is a suspected cause of cancer. Over the years, virally transmitted cancers also appear, e.g. herpes related viruses may be involved in the development of some forms of leukemia, Hodgkin's disease, cervical cancer and Burkett's lymphoma. It was also found that in some cases medical treatment increases a person's risk for cancer, e.g. hormonal therapy given to women to prevent miscarriage caused carcinoma cervix in their daughters.

A number of studies have claimed that social and psychological factors play a significant role in determining whether a person can get cancer. In an overview by Garssen (2002) twenty one studies were found investigated the role of psychological factors in initiation of cancer, while fifty studies examined the psychological factors in progression of cancer. Generally the reviews summarize stressful life events, social relationship, locus of control and personality factors coping and adjustment to illness, negative emotional states, psychiatric diagnosis and repression of negative emotions as causative and progression factors in cancer (Cwikel, Behar, Zabora, 1997; De Boer, Ryckman, Pruyn, Van den Borne, 1999). Stress has been implicated in increased susceptibility to several types of cancers. People, who are lonely, depressed and lack social support has been shown to be more susceptible to cancer than are their mentally healthy counterparts. The patients, who developed cancer, experienced a higher rate of stressful life events, before the onset of cancer. A feeling of hopelessness experienced in connection with a loss for which the person assumes personal responsibility, such as death of spouse increases the susceptibility to develop cancer (Sklar and Anisman, 1981)

The role of personality factors in development of cancer was also indicated in early researches, e.g. breast cancer was attributed to conflicts surrounding motherhood and femininity and to masochistic tendencies involving an inability to discharge negative emotions and unresolved hostility towards the mother. The idea of cancer-prone personality was also explored. A cancer-prone personality individual is characterized as easy going, and accepts things without any protest, repressing emotions that might interfere in smooth social and emotional functioning, trouble in expressing tension, anger or anxiety, instead presenting the self as pleasant, calm, compliant and passive and respond to stress with depression and hopelessness and develop learned helplessness. (Bahnson, 1981; Renneker, 1981; Temoshok, 1987). Kapoor, Ahmed and Ahmed (1987) compared cancer patients with normal subjects on the Indian adaptation of Cattle's 16 PF and found that cancer patients were significantly higher on anxiety, emotionality, sensitivity, depression, insecurity and tension as compared to their normal counterparts. Vaidya, Srivastava, and Srivastava (1985) compared cancer patients with hypertension patients and found that cancer patients were more dissatisfied with life, neurotic, unhappy and complaining people. Thus both overtly anxious and depressed, as well as, repressors who have trouble in expressing anxiety and anger have been linked to cancer. Besides these psychological factors, social factors like loss of support (Sklar and Anisman, 1981), absence of current social network (Thomas and Duszynski, 1974) absence of close family ties in childhood (Grassi and Mblinari, 1986) affect the onset and course of cancer. Kaplan and Reynolds (1988) found that women who were socially isolated were at significantly elevated risk of dying from cancer of all sites. Perhaps, social support and good healthy relationships have beneficial effects on emotional adjustment to the disease (Maunsell, Brisson, Deschenes, 1995). Personal support has positive relation to quality of life and partially mediates the effects of symptom distress (Manning-Walsh, 2005).

Studies have reported that cancer is influenced by psychological factors, and that both the onset and progression of the disease are affected by factors such as stress, depression, social isolation and coping style. Wonghongkal, Dechprom, Phumivichuvate and Losawatkul (2006) reported that uncertainty, and harm appraisal influence quality of life of breast cancer survivors. Social support plays a vital role in promoting overall QOL in breast cancer survivors (Lee, 1997). However, much of the research has been undermined by methodological weaknesses such as small sample size and failure to control for confounding factors (Edelman, in press).

Cardiovascular Diseases

Cardiovascular Diseases (CVDs) are diseases of the heart and blood vessels. CVDs also constitute a major chronic disease, which is a leading cause of death not only in India but all-over the world. There are many forms of cardiovascular diseases and many of them are interrelated. Some of the diseases are: (i) Atherosclerosis (Fatty plaque build-up in arteries), (ii) Heart attack (myocardial infraction), (iii) Chest pain (angina pectoris), (iv) Irregular heart beat (arrhythmia), (v) Congestive heart failure, (vi) Congenital and rheumatic heart disease and (vii) Stroke (cerebra vascular accident).

These diseases can be prevented or their course may be halted by taking certain steps to change in behaviour, diet and lifestyle, e.g. by maintaining weight, reducing saturated fats intake, decreasing sodium intake, regular exercising and changing lifestyle to reduce stress, give-up smoking.

Heart disease has family history component. It has been more common among the children of individuals who have had heart disease. The risk factors involved in heart diseases are high blood pressure, diabetes, cigarettes smoking, obesity, high serum cholesterol level and low level of physical activity (Criqui, 1986; Jeffery, 1992).

Besides the biological and heredity factors researchers have now found that the level of stress and one's method of coping with stress may influence the development of heart disease. Krantz and McCeney (2002) had reviewed the impact of psychological and psychosocial factors on the development and outcome of coronary heart disease, with particular emphasis on studies employing verifiable outcomes of CAD morbidity or mortality. Five key variables identified as possible psychosocial risk factors for CAD are: acute and chronic stress, hostility, depression, social support, and socio-economic status. Hostility, exposure to chronic stress and cardiovascular reactivity to stress contributes in the development of CHD. Brody (1993) found that acute stress, negative emotions and sudden bursts of activity can lead to sudden heart attack. Although stress may be a risk factor for coronary heart diseases, scientists still don't know exactly how stress might be involved in heart disease. But psychologists are agree that certain personality predispositions contribute either directly or indirectly to the etiology of particular forms of disease or to general illness susceptibility. For example: Type A behaviour syndrome is also identified as a psychological risk factor for cardiovascular disease. Type A behaviour (Friedman and Rosenman, 1974) was characterized by three components, easily aroused hostility, a sense of time urgency and competitive achievement strivings. Individuals displaying Type A behaviour pattern seem to be engaged in a ceaseless and often-fruitless struggle with themselves, with others, with circumstances and with time. Contrary to this Type B people are more relaxed, philosophical, cheerful and friendly. By the late 1970s, a sufficient body of evidences had been accumulated by biomedical and behavioural scientists to conclude that Type A behaviour is associated with increased risk for coronary heart disease independent of traditional CHD risk factors (Cooper, Detre and Weiss, 1981). In some studies depression, hostility anger, and low social support are associated with CAD, after controlling for adverse health behaviours, but not all studies (O'Malley, Jones,

Feuerstein and Taylor, 2000; Williams *et al.*, 2000) Contrary to common belief, Type A personality is not associated with an excess of CAD (Enas, 1996). Moreover, the prognosis of CAD among type A persons is better than in type B patients.

Some studies were conducted to examine the Type A behaviour pattern in India and the results of most of the Indian studies were similar to those found in the west. (e.g. Basu and Saha, 1985; Bhatia, Tiwari, Balkrishna and Gupta, 1990; Ghulam, Gupta, Bandyopadhyaya, and Mishra, 1990; Kaushik, Mukhopadhyaya, Sheik and Goel, 1991). Bhatia, Tiwari, Balkrishnan and Gupta (1990) interrogated MI patients within a week of hospitalization and noted Type A behaviour pattern in seventy two per cent of the CHD patients. Similarly, Kaushik, Mukhopadhyaya, Sheik and Goel (1991) found that for both male and female patients, Type A behaviour was an important precipitating factor. Researches have also suggested that not all behavioural components of the Type A behaviour syndrome increase the likelihood of CHD. Hostility, another dimension of Type A behaviour, is strongly implicated as a risk factor for CHD (Smith, 1992). Booth-Kewley and Friedman (1987) reviewed the literature and concluded that coronary proneness may be characterized more by chronic negative emotional states than by hurried, impatient workaholic Type A personality. Anxiety was also found a risk factor for CHD among women and men (Markowitz, *et al.* 1991). Similarly, extreme fatigue, a feeling of being dejected or defeated and an enhanced irritability also leads to CHD (Appel and Mulder, 1989; Appel and Otten, 1992). Expression of hostile emotions such as anger, and cynicism is associated with enhanced cardiovascular reactivity (Siegman, Anderson, Herbst, Boyle and Wilkinson 1992). Basu and Neogi (1999) compared the individuals suffering from cardiovascular diseases to those with normal healthy subjects and reported that normal subjects had greater ability to resolve life conflicts.

Depression appears to be a robust and prognostic cardiac risk factor associated with increased morbidity and mortality and complicates management of cardiac illness (Lenexa, Scott-Lenexa and Bohlig, 1993; Carney, *et al.*, 1987). Studies have documented that depression treatment in cardiac patients reduces symptoms and may decrease morbidity and disability, and improve quality of life (Nemeroff, Musselman, Evans, 1998; Patten, 1999). Besides, the personality related factors, the context in which individual live, negative events in his/her life, daily hassles and other such socio-cultural factors may also contribute to cardiovascular problems. Singh and Mishra (1987) studied thirty eight recently hospitalized Myocardial Infraction (MI) patients and found that death of a close family member, change in financial status and increased job responsibilities played an important role in the onset of MI.

Thus, a number of personality related variables, as well as, psychosocial variables have been studied in patients afflicted with coronary artery diseases. Some factors are important in exaggerating the complication of diseases but some others (like optimism, futurity, self-efficacy, less anxiousness, low hostility, etc.) reduces its stressful effect and push individuals to adjust with it and cope with it.

Diabetes

Diabetes is chronic disorder in which the body is not able to manufacture or properly utilize insulin. Insulin is the hormone secreted by the pancreas that controls the movement of glucose into cells and glucose metabolism. When there is an insulin dysfunction, there is an excess of glucose in the blood and this is discharged into the urine. Diabetes is of two types:

(a) Type I diabetes or insulin dependent diabetes which usually develops relatively early in the life, i.e., in childhood or adolescence and was formerly known as juvenile onset diabetes. It appears about 20 per cent of all types of diabetes.

(b) Type II diabetes or non-insulin dependent usually develops in adulthood. Many patients are essentially asymptomatic and most are overweight. Type II diabetic patients have retained some degree of endogenous insulin production; therefore, they are not dependent on exogenous insulin administration.

The diabetic is vulnerable to two blood sugar problems namely, hypoglycemia (a blood sugar level that is too low) and hyperglycemia (a blood sugar level that is too high). Hypoglycemia reaction is typically sudden but hyperglycemia is gradual medical intervention. Hyperglycemia appears to be directly related to the well-known heightened susceptibility of diabetes related infections. The most common site of infection in diabetic patients is the urinary tract. Other usual infections may occur predominantly in diabetics, e.g. invasive fungal infection of the nose and sinuses, invasive bacterial infection of the auditory canal. A trouble complication of hyperglycemia is abscesses and loss of teeth. Diabetics have to take great care for oral hygiene. Despite these potential problems with blood sugar level diabetic patients are more at risk because of the complications that develop due to it. Diabetes is associated with tightening of the arteries due to the building of wastes in the blood. As a result, diabetic patients show high rates of coronary heart disease. Diabetes is also the leading cause of blindness among adults, renal failure, difficulties in functioning such as eating disorders, impairment with memory etc. (Wing *et al*. 1986, Taylor and Rochman, 1988).

Diabetic foot ulcers are also very common and usually initiated by minor trauma but can become extensive, deep and spreading. Autonomic neuropathy is very troublesome and may occur in nearly one-third of all diabetic patients. Patients who are genetically predisposed to the development of hypertension may be especially at risk. The greatest risk to survival and quality of life of diabetic patients is the development of macro vascular atherosclerotic disease. Atherosclerosis and coronary artery disease have a considerably higher prevalence in diabetics than in non-diabetics of similar age group. The principal threat to the life of the diabetic patients is coronary artery disease. The incidence is high and mortality from an acute myocardial infraction is twice than in non-diabetics.

The basic goal of management of diabetes is the consistent maintenance of a normal blood glucose level. The cornerstone of long-term therapy is diet. Type II diabetic patients are usually obese. The objective of dietary management in these patients is weight reduction to ideal body weight. Saturated fat should be minimal because hyperlipidemia probably contributes to the excessively high incidence of vascular disease in these patients; frequent monitoring of the blood glucose is required for proper management of the patient. Diabetes management can be considered a balancing act between meeting the demands of the treatment and minimizing intrusion of treatment on everyday life.

The concept of quality of life offers a framework for understanding how individuals attempt to achieve this balance (Eiser and Tooke, 1995).

Diabetes is caused by any kind of damage to pancreas and insulin producing cells and there has been a suspicion that psychological factors predispose people to develop diabetes. It is, however, well researched that psychosocial factors play significant role after onset or diagnosis of the diabetes. Researchers have said that living with diabetes needs to be considered in a psychosocial context, because its treatment regimen is demanding and complex and patient has to adjust with it (Bradly and Marteau, 1986; Helz and Templeton, 1990). Gonder-Frederick and his colleagues (1990) stated that both Type I and Type II diabetics appear to be sensitive to the effects of stress. Stress adversely affects adherence and diet (Balfour, White, Schiffrin, Dougherty and Dufresne, 1993). Stress acts both directly and indirectly. Directly, it results in the production of pituitary hormones and catecholamine which results in increased blood sugar levels in both diabetics and non-diabetics. Indirectly, stress acts to change behaviour. These changes are likely to interfere with regimen adherence in a number of ways. Eating more or less when upset, forgetting to do blood tests or injections can occur. Stress has been seen as the cause of poor control. Poor control might interfere with general functioning, e.g. low blood sugar level may result in poor coping skills (Wales, 1995; Herpertz *et al.*, 2000).

Praming *et al.* (1986) highlights the difficulties that might occur during episodes of low blood sugar. The skills tested in this study were simple motor skills to complex memory and control and elapsed time estimation. Results showed that lowering in the blood sugar level below 3mmol/1 resulted in cognitive dysfunction in twelve out of sixteen subjects and when the levels dropped to less than 2mmol/l dysfunction in all subjects. The test showed gradual deterioration (except for simple psychomotor tests) and the deterioration was characterized by diminished attention.

Holmes (1986) stated that adaptation to each phase of diabetes is determined by individual's current circumstances and the emotions and perceptions these can evoke from past experiences. In some cases it was found that social support increases the likelihood of adhering treatment regimen and adjustment with diabetes but in other cases it did not happen, e.g. Kaplan and

Hartwell (1987) found that satisfaction with social support helped women diabetic patients maintain their complex diet chart and exercise routine, social support may also have beneficial effects on emotional adjustment to the disease. Littlefield, Rodin, Murray and Craven (1990) found that in patients with a number of illness related disabilities, availability of social support protected them from becoming depressed. Patients without a strong social support network were more likely to become depressed as their diabetes related disabilities progressed.

Family members are usually involved during the course of a chronic illness. Murphy, Williamson and Nease (1994) studied whether family participation was associated with the diabetic adults' level of metabolic control. A telephone survey of 131 diabetic adults was conducted. In the results two broad categories of family participation were found (i) Family Health Monitor (FHM) or internal health expert for family, (ii) distinct primary supportive family member or helper defined as family member who performs at least one supportive task in the care of the illness. Three-fourth of diabetic adults had identified on FHM in their families. Eighty seven per cent of FHM's were women, usually adult daughters of diabetic women or wives of diabetic men. The most frequent helping task involved dietary issues, medication, general support and blood sugar monitoring. Studies on family environment in glycemic control showed that when family members supported diabetes care regimen gave more satisfaction with adaptation to illness. Family cohesion also related to better physical function. Family system variables are related to psychosocial adaptation (Trief, Grant, Elbert and Weinstock, 1998).

Living with diabetes is not easy. It has been estimated that up to 75 per cent of the risk of type 2 diabetes is attributable to obesity. Recent clinical trials and observational epidemiologic studies demonstrate the efficacy of lifestyle changes, including decreased energy intake, decreased fat intake, and weight loss, as well as regular participation in physical activity, in improving insulin sensitivity and reducing the risk of diabetes (Costacou and Mayer-Davis, 2003). Adherence of dietary chart and maintenance of blood glucose to specified level is stress producing and difficult. Although individual differences are there, but several studies have demonstrated that in dealing with diabetes, psychosocial factors play a significant role.

Diabetes and Coronary Heart Disease

Diabetic patients are at greater risk of atherosclerosis and its clinical sequelae, particularly coronary artery disease. CAD remains the most important cause of mortality among diabetic patients. Hyperglycemia, insulin resistance, abnormal lipid profile, oxidative modification of lipoprotein, increased blood pressure etc. are the factors which accelerate the process of atherosclerosis in diabetic subjects. CAD in diabetic subjects carries a worse prognosis than in non-diabetic subjects. The risk for CAD in diabetic patients is 2 to 4 times as compared to their non-diabetic counterparts (Deepa, Arvind and Mohan, 2002; Uppaluri, 2002). There are evidences of strong association of diabetic and CAD in European and American population (Okosun, *et al.*, 2001; Sowers and Epstien, 1995). Silent myocardial ischemia occurs in greater than one in five asymptomatic patients with type 2 diabetes (Frans, *et al.*, 2004). Type 2 diabetes is associated with severe myocardial insulin resistance regardless of CAD and despite normal basal blood flow (Iozzo, 2002). Ohtake *et al.* (1995) reported insulin-stimulated glucose uptake to be slightly impaired in patients with type 2 diabetes without CAD. This finding was confirmed by Yokoyama *et al.* (2000). Similarly, Voipio-Pulkki *et al.* (1993) described the occurrence of the same phenomenon in type II diabetic patients. Asian Indians with diabetes and heart disease have a bad outlook; the immediate mortality is high and the complications are more frequent and often grave (Jarret, 1989). Khare, Raman, Bhatanagar and Bhavsar (2000) found the overall prevalence of vascular complications in diabetic subjects was high and considerably higher than that usually found in non-diabetic subjects. Diabetes could lead to asymptomatic coronary artery disease, hence as a preventive measure it is necessary for all diabetics above the age of 40 years to undergo stress ECG. It needs to be reinforced that an assessment of risk factors and their management like the control of body weight, lipids, blood pressure and smoking is more significant than mere control of blood glucose in such a situation. Even in the absence of well established risk factors of coronary artery disease, diabetes by itself is a significant contributor to this disease.

Psychosocial Factors in Chronic Illnesses

Chronic illness is stressful because this condition may never go away and can disrupt the lifestyle in many ways. Stress can build and influence how one feels about life. Prolonged stress can lead to frustration, anger, hopelessness and at times depression. The person with the illness is not the only one affected, family members are also affected by the persistent health changes of a loved one. Chronic illnesses are particularly stressful because a number of stressors attack the afflicted person at the same time. Some of these are: Chronic illness, uncertainty about future, unpredictability of disease, disability, financial difficulties, tough treatment regimen, adjustment difficulties, family problems etc.

Learning to manage stress will help the person to maintain a positive physical, emotional and spiritual outlook on life. The afflicted person must learn how to live with the physical effects of the illness, deal with treatment procedures, maintain emotional balance to cope with negative feelings, maintain confidence and positive self-images, maintain trust and confidence in the doctor, maintain social relationships, avoid social isolation, understand the condition, know how to control the symptoms. The diagnosis of any chronic illness confronts individuals with a collection of tasks necessary for both physical and psychological adjustment. Adjustment may involve acceptance of a certain amount of loss of function. Acceptance does not mean the person is surrendering to illness and does not go for treatment but it does mean that he has accepted the reality that he has to make certain changes in his life-style to be a fully functioning man even with this long-term illnesses. It may also require the acquisition of new skills and changes to daily routines in order for the patient to manage the symptoms of the illness or cope with the demands of treatment. As such, chronic illness places a considerable burden on the individual and can have a significant impact on their quality of life. From earlier researches, it is clear that the illness perceptions of individuals are highly influential in determining outcomes and adjustment in a number of medical conditions.

The centre of wellness lies in the concept of adaptation and creative use of resources to maximize choices. Positive self-esteem is needed for true adaptation and to be psychologically well while suffering from physical illness. Illness leads to both emotional, as well as, physical upheaval. How people will react to illness depends on many conditions, e.g. the severity of illness (The very sick person put all their energy into healing and fighting with the disease and may not have the luxury of energy left over for emotional growth), the kind of social support available, the pre-illness personality and psychological resources of the person. The diagnosis, duration of disease and developmental stage of the patient's children were useful in predicting the impact of chronic illness on patient's physical functioning. Diagnosis, duration of disease, and economic status had a significant impact on a patient's psychological functioning. Diagnosis, age, mental status, the developmental stage of the children and the primary caregiver were the most important factors related to the effects of chronic illness on adults (Hwu, 1995).

Hope is an important strategy in coping with chronic illnesses (Raleigh, 1992). In his study he found that family, friends and religious beliefs were most commonly reported sources for supporting hopefulness. Patients were able to identify specific ways in which these sources helped to support their hope. The majority of patients reported positive attitudes about their illnesses, with transient periods of lowered hope. Studies have supported the view that recovery from chronic illness is possible. Disorbio and his associates (1991) identified factors that influenced recovery from chronic illness. Using a computerized test battery, they demonstrated how psychosocial and lifestyle factors affected recovery. In the light of this frightening and disturbing scenario of prevalence of chronic diseases, it is worthwhile to understand the psychological and social factors which may help in happy living and survival of the chronically ill patients. Review of literature suggests that psychological factors or personal characteristics of the individual may be helpful in overcoming the effect of stressors, like, loss of job or spouse or break in relationship or chronic illness etc. Some studies show that optimism was found to be associated with increased present life satisfaction, future life satisfaction and less negative mood (Curbow *et al.* 1993). Findings from this review indicate that support from parents (especially the mother) and friends were extremely important and that the adolescents were satisfied with family support. Support from friends was described as less satisfactory.

Chronic illness condition affects not only the relative medical status of individual, but the entire family's social life, emotional stability, financial resources and psychological health (Burish and Bradly, 1983; Taylor and Aspinwell, 1990). Just after the diagnosis of chronic disease, patients are often in a state of physical, mental and psychological disequilibrium (Moos, 1977). Generally, anxiety, fear, depression, denial, feeling of disorganization may be experienced (Taylor and Aspinwell, 1990) and their habitual ways of coping with problems go in vain. Researchers have argued that for successful and well adjusted living with chronic illness condition, it is very essential to understand the chronic condition and associated factors in psychosocial context. The role of a number of psychological characteristics like, optimism (Agarwal and Pandey, 1998; Agarwal and Tripathi, 2000), explanatory style (Peterson, Seligman and Valliant, 1988), hope (Snyder, 1994), hardiness (Kobassa, 1979), perceived control (Taylor *et al.*, 1991), happiness (Diener, 1994), positive illusions (Taylor, 1983), finding meaning in a traumatic event (Affleck, Tennen, Croog and Levine, 1987), negative affectivity (Costa and McCare, 1984), depression (Rodin and Vorshart, 1986; Primeau, 1986), anxiety (e.g. Grayden, 1988; Carey and Burish, 1985), hostility (McCare and Costa, 1984) and so many others have been examined. Psychologists repeatedly stated that these psychosocial factors become especially important under the challenging and life threatening circumstances.

In the present piece of work psychological characteristics of optimism, future orientation, perceived control and symptoms reported in patients suffering from chronic diseases, were investigated. Social factor, like, family environment was also studied because in earlier studies these psychosocial variables have been found to moderate responses to illness related stress.

Future Orientation

One of the advantages, which human beings enjoy, is that they can think of past, present and future at the same time. Psychologists have investigated this ability and have given concepts, like, time perspective, time orientation, future orientation, time management etc. The concept of psychological time perspective includes the total mental representation of past, present and future. Frank (1939) introduced the concept of "time perspective" in order to give psychological explanation of individuals concerning time. Lewin (1948) had adopted this concept into his Field theory of personality to define life space.

Future orientation is concerned with only one aspect of time, i.e. future (Lewin 1948), whereas, psychological past and present are also included in time perspective. Lewin (1948) had defined future orientation as a component which is comprised of "plans, aspirations, expectations and fears concerning events and actions realistically possible in the near or distant future."

This definition of future orientation implies that all types of future events consists of two components (i) a cognitive component corresponding to the subjective probabilities attached to the events and (ii) a motivational component that consists of the value that the events carry. Some researchers (e.g. Nuttin, 1964; Lessing, 1972) have emphasized the necessity of considering the motivational aspect of future orientation when trying to explain individual behaviour.

Future orientation has usually been analyzed by the length of future time perceived by the individual. In cognitive aspect of future orientation the type (content) and the number of concerns (density) was also measured. A less structured future orientation can imply that the person has little interest in his future. He is not much concerned about his future. Besides this another aspect of future orientation is the way in which a person anticipates the causes of possible developments in future and the reasons behind these particular developments, e.g. using attribution theory whether she/he believes in the internal or external factors or stable or unstable factors.

The motivational aspect of future orientation is the anticipation of instrumental acts to attain positive and to avoid negative future developments. The researchers working in this area believe that the motivational and affective aspects of future orientation must be studied because these are important from the point of view of behavioural relevance of future orientation. According to decision making theory (Solvic *et al.*, 1977) the future is like a mirror of the past (Kates, 1962) with anticipation of future derived from past experiences. This would imply that positive experiences further a more optimistic future orientation than negative experiences.

The researches on time perspective and future orientation were concerned with the socio-psychological conditions of time perspective and future orientation and its behavioural consequences. The concept of time perspective and future orientation developed in a child just like a number of other concepts such as space, colures etc., and is influenced by a number of variables, like, family, age, social relations, gender etc. The early period of life a child places events in time on the basis of personal experiences but gradually this perception is influenced by external factors (Klineberg, 1967) and with the advancement of age it become more complex (Agarwal and Tripathi, 1984).

In a study featuring the development of knowledge of time of future events in children Friedman (2000) demonstrated that 4 year old children failed to differentiate future distances, 5 year olds were able to distinguish events that would occur in the coming weeks and months from those that would not occur for many months, 6 to 8 years of age made differentiate distances of events more than a few months in the future. By 8 to 10 years of age children accurately judged distances by using representations of the times of events in the annual cycle. Agarwal (2003) also reported that future orientation increases from childhood to adulthood. But this increment is not in a linear form. Future orientation sometimes decreases or remains stable during adolescence.

Earlier Trommsddorff (1978) established through empirical findings that experiences transmitted via family and school result in differences in future orientation. Sex and education determine personal planning, goal setting, hopes and fears. Future orientation, however, does not remain stable throughout life. Job experiences are much more real than school experiences as it challenges more personal interests, goals and desires.

Findings have suggested that judgment of future started in late childhood. Psychologists are also interested in knowing the age and gender differences in anticipation of future. Fingerman and Perlmutter (1995) examined the age differences in future time perspective, locus of control and past and anticipated future life events in two groups of men and women, a younger group (aged between 20 to 37 years) and an older group (aged between 60 to 81 years). Results showed that there were no age and gender differences in the time period about which participants thought most frequently. It was, however, reported that younger group of participants thought frequently about more distant time periods.

Besides the examination of age and gender differences in future orientation, several empirical studies were conducted to know the correlates of future time perspective in different groups of people, like, adolescents, adults, elderly, students, patients, victims of war and accidents, deprived, institutionalized etc. For example: Agrawal (2003), Agrawal, Tripathi and Srivastava (1983) studied the influence of socio-cultural factors on time perspective in deprived groups. They found that deprivation reduces the tendency to think and plan about future. These investigators also studied the relationship of time perspective, reflectivity, impulsively and delay of gratification. The results showed that reflective style positively affects future orientation and helps a person tolerate the delay in getting rewards.

Studies on students' future time perspective and its correlates particularly indicated the motivational consequences of time perspective. Murrel and Mingrone (1994) found that individuals with an orientation towards future time placed strong emphasis on success through goal directed behaviour. They pay more attention to cues existing in the environment and engage themselves in a large number of activities to achieve the goals they set for themselves. Similarly, Shell and Huesman (2001) investigated the relations between college students control beliefs and future time perspective and their academic achievement. They used canonical correlations and found that future time perspective is associated with grades achieved by students. Future time perspective beliefs play role in motivating achievement and studying.

Review of literature on time perspective suggests that numerous studies had been conducted to understand its role in aging. The data particularly showed that older adults are at risk of developing a less extended and less personal future (Rakowski, 1979). Lomranz *et al.*, (1985) also reported that the tendency to rate past events increases with the progress of age, whereas, the future ratings decreases. Shmotkin (1991) surveyed Israeli elderly population and reported that with the advancement of age, ratings for future had declined, a mild decline in ratings for present and ratings for past had a relative increase. The ratings of present trend to remain stable across the life-span. Steverink and Kempen (1998) stated that certainly age has an influence on future time perspective of elderly, but resources (like competence belief, social contact and affection) play a relatively larger role than age. Empirical evidences suggest that in elderly population past, as well as, present is salient but thinking and planning about future faces a decline. Generally in elderly people the goal set for them are fulfilled, so attention on time perspective also declines.

A good amount of work had been done to understand the role of future orientation in encouraging preventive health behaviour, health education and experiences of chronic illness. Rothspan and Read (1996) examined the present versus future time perspective among college students. They hypothesized that safer sex behaviours might reduce the exposure to HIV would positively correlate with future orientation. In the results, it was found that high future oriented were less likely to be sexually experienced and had fewer sexual partners. Highly future oriented students were more likely to use alternate methods of reducing exposure to HIV. This study shows that future oriented outlook enhances preventive behaviours.

Since future orientation is associated with preventive behaviours it is pertinent to ask whether it leads to well-being and happiness. A number of studies which have investigated this and other related questions have been reviewed. Misra and Agarwal (2003) found that future orientation had significant positive association, with women's possession of social skills and better psychological well-being. Women who have more structured future time perspective were more satisfied and happy with their lives. Wenseuier and Grossmen (1998) studied attachment representation, subjective life satisfaction and future time perception in elderly people. Their results showed that elderly participants with secure attachment representation were more satisfied, less anxious and more positive about their future. Both of these studies showed that future orientation is a predictor of well-being, as well as, outcome of it. Lang and Carstensen (2002) tried to examine the extent to which future time perspective is related to social motivation and perceived quality of personal network in a group of participants age ranged between 20 to 90 years. In general, they found that older people perceived their future as more limited than younger group. Those who perceived future as bleak and limited had given priority to emotionally meaningful goals and this was found to be associated with greater social satisfaction. Perceived quality of personal network was dependent on future time perspective.

Generally studies on aging and illness suggest that aged persons are predominantly present time oriented. Aged and chronically ill patients have some commonality. The physical functioning of both have been limited, constraints in doing daily routine work, more and more engagement in health maintenance behaviours etc. Lennings (2000) said the extent to which the elderly perceive or value the future may have an impact on health enhancing behaviours. Optimism increases with age but satisfaction decreases with age. Lennings argued that decrement in satisfaction is related more to a sense of realism about the tasks related with aging than a sense of "death anxiety" or avoidance of future. Upadhyay (2002) examined influence of optimism, future orientation and detachment on health and recovery of operated patients and their healthy counterparts. She found that future orientation predicted lower scores on negative mental state questionnaire in surgical patients, as well as, in total group. Optimistic personal control and detached future predicted recovery from surgery. Quality of life was also predicted by future orientation.

Reviewing the relationship between future orientation and well-being, it can be said that thinking and planning about future or looking at future in a more positive way enhances the health maintenance behaviour and overall well-being. Chronic illness involves the patient in a process of assessing his health status, strength and weaknesses. This kind of health experience along with the person's global orientation towards future may affect the process of coping. Pandey and Agrawal (1998) examined the future orientation in coping with chronic diseases and found significant differences between highly future oriented and low future oriented groups in the use of mental disengagement, active coping, acceptance, positive reinterpretation, denial and seeking instrumental social support coping strategies. In general, high future oriented participants used more positive and problem focused coping strategies as compared with low future oriented participants.

Wills, Sandy and Yaeger (2001) investigated the relation of time perspective to early onset substance use in a sample of elementary school students. Results revealed that future orientation negatively related to substance use and the relation of times perspective was mediated through behavioural coping and coping with anger. Role of future orientation in coping process was examined in another context by Misra and Agarwal (2003). They studied this relationship in working and non-working women. Here again it was found that future orientation was positively related with active coping, planning and restraint coping.

Thus, future orientation had been studied in different contexts and it has an important role in coping with adverse situation of any kind. Although elderly people have a less extended future outlook in general but those who realistically think about future are well adjusted and active copers.

Dispositional Optimism

Power of positive thinking has been identified by researchers for decades. The common view is that positive thinking can help a person to overcome from adversity, recover from long-term illness, help in attainment of goals and help in succeeding and removing the obstacles (Cousin, 1977; Peale, 1956). Historically, Optimism appears to be positive asset. Valtaire, in Candida stated that "Optimism is a mania for maintaining that all is well when things are going badly." Similarly, James Cabell, in the Silver Stalion said, "The optimist proclaims that live in the best of all possible worlds and the pessimist fears that this is true."

In contemporary world of psychology the concept of "dispositional optimism" has been investigated in detail and established by Scheier and Carver (1985). They suggested that dispositional optimism may have important implications for the manner in which people deal with the life's stresses (Scheier and Carver, 1987; Reker and Wong, 1985). Scheier and Carver (1985) defined optimists as people who "expect things to go their way and generally believe that good rather than bad things will happen to them."

The concept of optimism and pessimism has attracted the researchers in the fields of personality, social, clinical and health psychology over past few decades (e.g. Aspinwell and Taylor, 1992, 1997; Chang, 1996; Cozzarelli, 1983; Fischer and Leitchberg 1986; Norem and Cantor, 1986; Peterson, Seligman and Valliant, 1988; Weinstein, 1980). Empirical investigations of optimism as an individual difference witnessed that optimism is a highly beneficial psychological characteristic found to be linked to good mood, perseverance, achievement, and physical health. Optimism was associated with better mood, higher numbers of helper T cells, and higher natural killer cell cytotoxicity (Peterson, 2000).

The concept of optimism was not a new one. It has its roots in theoretical model of behavioural self-regulation (e.g. Carver and Scheier, 1981, 1983, 1985). This model assumes that expectations of successful outcomes cause people to renew their efforts to attain and set goals, if and when disruption of goal directed activities occur. If expectancies are sufficiently unfavourable, the result is reduced vigour or even a complete disengagement from further goal-directed effort (e.g. Bandura, 1977, Feather, 1982). Tiger (1979) strongly stated that optimism is an inherent part of human nature and one of the most defining and adaptive characteristics of human being. Optimism is developing along with the cognitive abilities and human capacity for culture.

Lazarus, Beck, Taylor and some other psychologists described optimism to speculate individual differences. It was said that the nature of human being provides baseline optimism, on the basis of this people show more or less optimism. Researches have indicated that optimism linked with happiness, perseverance, achievement and health. Scheier, Carver, Peterson, Seligman in a number of studies inquired into the relationship between optimism and other variables like health, happiness, well-being and coping with crisis and found that dispositional optimism is linked to desirable outcomes.

In one of the earlier studies Reker and Wong (1983) studied a group of institutionalized and non-institutionalized elderly persons and found that persons who were earlier assessed as optimists reported fewer symptoms at the time of two year follow-up along with positive physical, psychological and general well-being. Carver and Gains (1987) investigated the effect of dispositional optimism on emotional well-being on a group of mothers of newly born babies. The women have completed dispositional optimism and depression in the last trimester of their pregnancy and then 3 weeks after the birth of their babies. Results revealed that optimism predicted lower levels of depressive symptoms postpartum, even when controlling for initial levels. One of the pioneers in the area of studying optimism, Scheier and Carver explored the role of optimism in a wide variety of situations, including optimistic orientation of students before examination, surgical patients and chronically ill patients. Scheier *et al.* (1989) inspected subjective reactions and recovery pattern of patients' months later. Dispositional optimism, coping strategies, mood, perceived recovery and quality of life were assessed and also other medical data were gathered. Results revealed that before surgery optimists had less hostility and depression than pessimists. One week after surgery optimists said feeling of relief and more happiness, satisfaction with their medical care and more satisfaction with emotional support from friends. Six months later optimists reported higher quality of life as compared to pessimists. In a 5 years follow-up on these same patients' optimism continued to be the most important prospective predictor of subjective well-being and better and better quality of life. Carver *et al.* (1993) studied the psychological adaptation to treatment for early stage breast cancer in women. Patients were interviewed at three stages, at the time of diagnosis, on the day prior to surgery and 7 to 10 days after surgery. Follow-up interview were conducted 3, 6, and 12 months later. Dispositional optimism predicted not just lower initial distress but also resilience against distress during the year follow-up surgery. Pessimism places patients at risk for adverse outcomes in several respects, rather than solely with regard to emotional distress (Carver, Lehman, Antoni, 2003). Cozzarelli (1993) examined the influences of optimism on adjustment to abortion and found that optimism was related to psychological adjustment. Given *et al.* (1993) studied a group of cancer patients and their caregivers and it was found that optimism not only positively influences psychological well-being of patients with medical problems but also have an impact on well-being of caregivers. Hooker *et al.* (1992), Shifren and Hooker (1995) also found similar results.

Bedsides these studies the long-term significance of optimism pessimism was also investigated. In a longitudinal prospective study Peterson *et al.* (1988) found that pessimism at age 25 was significantly associated with poorer psychological and physical adjustment 25 years later. This classic study suggests that optimistic outlook or always looking for brighter side is not only important for present adjustment but also valuable for adjustment in future.

Thus reviewing literature related to optimism and well-being, it is apparent that optimism is a positive characteristic, which leads to good psychosocial adjustment and perception of satisfaction and happiness in all respects. Particularly, those studies which examined this relationship in the context of chronic illnesses, demonstrated that remains optimistic in such a life threatening condition, reduces the perception of severity of threat and increases the vigour to fight with the disease.

Dispositional optimism, conceptualized as the generalized expectancy for positive outcomes, has been found to account for individual differences in psychological and physical well-being. It has also been linked to the use of different coping strategies in the wake of adversity. The relationship between optimism and coping was examined in a longitudinal study on a group of men at risk for AIDS by Taylor *et al.* (1992), and found that optimists scored higher on maintaining positive attitudes as a coping strategy and lower on the fatalism/self-blame and escape than pessimists. Taylor *et al.* (1992) also found that optimism was related with active coping strategies. In their study on coronary artery bypass surgery patients Scheier *et al.* (1989) found that before surgery optimists were making plans for their future and setting goals for their recovery. One week after surgery optimists were seeking more information than pessimists from their doctors about what they had to do in coming months. Optimists were also not suppressing thoughts about their physical symptoms. These results suggest that optimists not only engaged in active problem focused coping strategies but they are more realistic towards their condition. Litt *et al.* (1992) examined coping in a study on individuals who had failed *in vitro* fertilization. Optimists reported that they had benefited somehow from this experience and became closer to their spouse. Thus optimists see a silver line in clouds. Stanon and Snider (1993) studied on women going for breast biopsy. They assessed the optimism, mood and coping of women a day before biopsy. Those women who were diagnosed with a non-malignant cancer completed a second assessment. Women with pessimistic outlook used more cognitive avoidance coping before the upcoming diagnostic procedure than did optimists. Among women with positive diagnosis cognitive avoidance before the biopsy predicted post-biopsy distress. On the other hand, optimists use active coping strategy (Misra and Agarwal, 2003).

Studies show that optimism leads to the use of more active problem focused coping strategies not only in chronic, life threatening health conditions but also to terminal health conditions. Park, Moore, Turner and Adler (1997) studied the adjustment of women to their pregnancy and found that optimist women were more engaged in constructive thinking. Constructive thinking was defined as a tendency to think about and solve daily problems in an effective manner.

In nutshell, the results of the studies on optimism and coping conclude that optimists differ from pessimists in their use of coping strategies. Optimists use more problems focused coping strategies than do pessimists. When they found difficulty in using problem focused coping strategies, they turn to strategies such as acceptance, use of humour and positive reframing. Acceptance keeps the person goal-engaged and indeed life-engaged (Carver and Scheier, 1998; Scheier and Carver, 2001)

Perceived Control

Perceived control refers to a person's self-assessment of control one has on various aspects of his life, the ways and means to acquire expected outcomes and also to avoid unexpected ones. To have a sense of control has become especially important in adverse situations where such a positive focus to find a meaning in life leads to enhanced quality of life and use of effective coping strategies.

Several theorists have emphasized the importance of perception of control, and stated that it is the fundamental characteristic of human beings to control the world around us (Schultz *et al.*, 1994). Those theorists who do not agree that this is the root of desire to control in evolutionary framework suggested that control drive is the central motivation guiding human behaviour and development (White, 1959). Thompson and Wierson (2000) stated that generally individuals use three strategies to maintain control even is awesome circumstances. These are: (i) Changing to goals that are reachable in current circumstances. (ii) Creating new avenues for control, and (iii) Accepting current circumstances.

Generalized beliefs about control were studied in a variety of situations. Most of the researches in the relationship between stress and control are based on the assumption that having a sense of control is stress reducing and not having a sense of control is stress inducing. Steptoe (1989) had described the significance of perceived control and said that most of the health related researches have especially focused on the control over aversive stimulation and on conditions in which the goal of control is the elimination of aversive events.

Control-related beliefs become important in the context of threatening traumatic events. Several investigations revealed that when individuals have sustained a traumatic health event, they come to believe that they have control over at least some aspects of that event. In studies with breast cancer patients (Taylor *et al.*, 1984), men with AIDS (Reed *et al.*, 1993) and heart disease patients (Taylor, Helgenson *et al.*, 1991), data revealed that the majority of patients felt that they had at least some or a high degree of control over their disease. These beliefs appear to be moderated by one's state of illness or prognosis. Thus, for example, asymptomatic breast cancer patients often assert that they have control over the disease itself and can prevent it from coming back (Taylor *et al.*, 1984), whereas, men in the advanced stages of AIDS regard themselves as having a high degree of control over their day-to-day medical care and treatment, but only some degree of control over their overall course of illness. People high in feelings of perceived control are less likely to appraise events as threatening or negative. Patients who believe they can control illness are better off than those who do not see their illness as under their control. They may believe that they can prevent a recurrence of disease through good health habits or by will-power or by complying with the treatment regimen. Evidences have suggested that feelings of psychological control may be beneficial for good mental functioning. Persons who feel that they have some control over their lives may be better adjusted than those who feel that they have no control on their lives. Taylor *et al.* (1984a) found that those cancer patients who believed that they had control over their illness were better adjusted to their cancer than patients without such beliefs. Similar results have been obtained for patients suffering from rheumatoid arthritis (Affleck, Tennen, Pfeiffer and Fifield, 1987; Tennen *et al.*, 1992) and post myocardial infraction patients (Helgenson, 1992). Bar-On (1986, 1987) studied the patients recovering from myocardial infraction and illustrated the importance of both causal attributions for illness and feelings of MI patients. Those patients, who attributed the cause of their MI to modifiable factors under their personal control such as stress or smoking, were more likely to have initiated active plans for their activities. The results of this study suggest that when illness conditions are perceived as being modifiable and under one's personal control, the process of recovery from chronic disease is enhanced. The model suggests that developing an internal locus of control would enhance the effectiveness of living with diabetes (Madhu, Veena and Sridhar, 1997).

The relationship between controllability and coping has been studied in several ways. Several investigators have suggested that generalized beliefs about control and situational control appraisals are related to coping efforts and persistence. Strikland (1978) reviewed the researches on internal-external locus of control and noted that studies indicated that people with internal locus of control are more likely to engage in an information search about disease and health maintenance when it is relevant for well-being. A person might be expected to control one aspect of a situation but not another. Silver and Wortman (1980b) studied the patients with spinal cord injuries and pointed out that one patient may believe that learning to get in and out of a bed to the wheelchair is in his control but being able to walk again is only in the control of God. The role of perceived control in coping with stressful life circumstances (Taylor, 1983) and the deficits associated with lack of control (Seligman, 1975) have been emphasized in literature. Having a sense of control is found to be associated with better coping with stressful life events (Glass, McKnight and Valdimarsdottir, 1993; Litt, 1988). Perception of control enhances problem solving and attention to solutions. People with strong sense of control are more likely to determine the cause of their problem than the people with a weak sense of control. It was reported that those with a low sense of control tend to use more the ineffective coping strategy of avoiding the problem. Perception of control is beneficial because it allows the person to prepare for an upcoming stress and ensure that the situation will not become intolerable (Miller, 1979). Brandsteadter and Rothermund (1994) studied the older adults and reported that by de-emphasizing the importance of unattainable goals and focusing on more reachable goals older adults maintain a strong sense of control.

Rothbaum, Weisz and Snyder (1982) had done a distinction between primary and secondary control. Primary control is the perception that one can get desired outcome and secondary control is accepting one's life circumstances as they are. Acceptance increases a sense of control because it helps people feel less helpless victims and reduces the discrepancy between desired and achieved outcome. Griffin and Rabkin (1998), Thompson, Nanni and Levine (1994) found that people with a greater sense of perceived control are less anxious and depressed in the face of chronic illnesses. Those with a stronger sense of perceived control are more likely to take needed action to improve or protect their physical health (Peterson and Stunkard, 1989; Robin, 1986), and also they have generally a better health status (England and Evans, 1992).

Researches have identified that in almost every sphere of life, a sense of perceived control has positive implications on emotional, physical, psychological and general well-being. Although sense of perceived control has been found as a positive characteristic in dealing with stress but cultural differences are also significant. Sastry and Ross (1998) examined the relationship between Asian culture and sense of control and impact of perceived control on depression and anxiety among Asians and non-Asians. Findings suggested Asians have lower levels of perceived control than non-Asians. High levels of perceived control were associated less strongly with psychological well-being in the case of Asians. They have interpreted these findings in terms of collectivist values in Asia. In contrary to individualistic western cultures, Asian cultures emphasis selfless subordination to family and community which may reduce levels of personal control. It has been assumed that the dictates of collectivist cultures are such that high levels of personal control among Asians may be perceived as a norm violation. Warr (1987) identified nine Principal Environmental Influences (PEI) or environmental categories which acting in conjunction with person factors, facilitate or constrain psychological well-being or mental health. These are: opportunities for control, opportunity for skill use, externally generated goals, variety, environmental clarity, availability of money, physical security, opportunity for interpersonal contact and valued social position. Of all the environmental influences, the intrinsic PEI opportunity for control is assumed to be the principal "foundation of mental health".

Review of literature show that perception of control is advantageous. Particularly, for the people who have struck with some traumatic life threatening disease. It may prompt individuals to take necessary actions. It activates problem solving and concentrates the person to seek the pathways of solution. Thus, it is pertinent to study this important variable in Indian socio-cultural context.

Symptoms Reported

Health professionals are gradually accepting that along with physical and physiological factors, psychological variables and personality of the individual may also influence the perception of health and illness and also the reporting of physical symptoms (Costa and McCrae, 1985; Pennebaker, 1982; Watson and Pennebaker, 1989). Commonly, reported symptoms (physical or psychological), by patients to the physician are used as the major primary criterion for disease. Patient presents a list of symptoms to the physician and accordingly the practitioner makes a diagnosis and then pathological tests and other investigations are carried out in order to make final diagnosis. This is the objective criterion of disease (Cohen, Tyrell and Smith, 1991; Macintyre and Pritchard, 1989). But the degree of correspondence between subjective and objective criteria is a matter of research. Feldman *et al.*, (1999) found that self-report is moderately associated with the objective disease criteria and there are personality characteristics and psychological processes that contribute to the perception of symptoms and illness. The identification of factors that influence physical and psychological symptoms reporting is important. A large number of individuals, who seek medical care, make somatic complaints which are not attributable to organic causes (Lepowski, 1988). Although illness reporting is expected to follow from the perception of physical symptoms, illness reporting may also depend on psychological processes as well (Cohen and Williconson, 1991).

Personality factors are widely researched in the context of perception and reporting of symptoms (Costa and McCrae, 1985, Pennebaker, 1982; Watson and Pennebaker, 1989). Perception of symptoms encourages one to define oneself as ill. Wiebe and Smith (1997) said that in reporting of illness, personality characteristics are linked to symptoms reporting. Neuroticism is one such personality factor which is widely researched for the evidence of personality biases in symptoms reporting (Costa and McCrae, 1987;

Watson and Pennebaker, 1989). The studies on neuroticism generally showed that neuroticism is related to reporting more frequent and severe symptoms and reporting more symptoms is independent of actual disease course. Studies with diabetic patients show that neuroticism is associated with a propensity to report more medically unexplained symptoms, symptoms related to hypoglycemia, worry about hypoglycemia and severe physical and emotional problems related to diabetes (Deary, Clyde and Frier, 1997; Deary and Frier, 1995; Hepburn, Deary, Madeod and Frier, 1994). Costa (1987), Shekelle, Venson and Ostfeld (1991) found that neuroticism is prospectively related to angina pectoris but not to objective signs of coronary artery disease. Skelton and Pennebaker (1978) found that Type A individuals are more prone than Type B in reporting symptoms. Personality characteristics of introversion-extraversion are also found to be associated with greater physiological responsiveness to pain (Stelmack, 1990). Extroverted individuals, who suffer from chronic pain, are more likely to report pain symptoms than introverted individuals (Harkins, Price and Braith, 1989).

In spite of the evidences that personality characteristics contribute to perception of symptoms and symptoms reporting situational factors, like, stress may contribute in symptoms reporting. People under stressful conditions report more and severe symptoms. Salovery *et al.* (1991) found that people who were in positive mood, reported fewer illness related memories and symptoms. Recognition of symptoms is determined by both individual differences and situational factors.

Evidences suggest that greater number of psychological and physical symptom reporting negatively affect the quality of life. Luscombe (2003) studied sufferers of irritable bowel syndrome. This syndrome was diagnosed through symptoms such as abdominal pain and irregular bowel habits. These symptoms plus the influence of psychological factors and extra intestinal symptoms adversely affect the health related quality of life of individuals. Von Dras and Lichty (1990) studied the symptoms and well-being in relation to glycemic control in Type II diabetes in 188 patients between 40 and 75 years. A cross-sectional relation between glycemic control and physical symptoms showed that glycemic control in Type II diabetes was associated with fewer physical symptoms, better mood and better well-being. Dazord *et al*. (1994) examined the depressive symptoms reporting and well-being of hundred patients with Type I diabetes. Women patients had a tendency to report more depressive symptoms and this leads to lowered well-being as compared with men. Patients with better professional activity had better perception of well-being. Results also indicated that the higher the level of anxiety and depression, lower the energy and positive feelings. Well-being improved with better glycemic control.

Well-being and symptoms of illness are inversely correlated. Evidences suggest that illness makes people less happy (Okum, Stock, Haring and Witter, 1984). Other studies, however, suggest that the inverse relation between self-reported health (in the form of complaining about symptoms) and subjective well-being results primarily from unhappy people perceiving more symptoms of illness.

Generally it appeared that symptoms reported by patients reflect the patients' levels of anxiety and depression and the presence of psychological illness (Trew and Maguire, 1982). Now, the question is how it is related with coping strategies, Rothrock, Lutegendort and Kreder (2003) studied coping strategies in patients with interstitial cystitis and the relationship of coping strategies with quality of life and depression. They found greater venting was associated with greater depressive symptoms and poorer mental health. Seeking instrumental social support was associated with depressive symptoms reporting. These findings suggest that maladaptive coping strategies were associated with higher levels of depressive symptoms and quality of life decrement in patients.

Several studies have shown that individuals with chronic back pain who have coping style characterized by passivity, avoidance or excessive negativity show heightened levels of depressive symptoms (Turner and Clancy, 1986). Similar finding have been reported in individuals with multiple sclerosis (Sullivan, Edgley *et al*., 1992). It can be concluded that symptoms are important and interesting indicators of physical and psychological experiences. They represent the complaints people have. Symptoms reporting are very common and used in general conversations by people about the stressors and strains of modern living. Symptoms reporting reflect the cognitive representation of illness as perceived by people. It is, therefore, important to understood symptom reporting behaviour and its role in coping and well-being.

Family Environment

A family is an organization of people who interact with one another and influence one another in many ways. People live in families particularly for seeking love, affection and emotional security. The number of functions a family might perform is unlimited and this is the unique characteristic of a family that its field of action is not strictly defined. As the new circumstances emerges the family can specify new roles, duties, rights and actions, as needed. The role of family as a significant support system became much more important when a crisis struck, e.g., the onset of a chronic illness like, cancer, diabetes or CHD to a family member, is such a problem that may get started through a crisis which is irresolvable. The families have to live with such difficulties that continue a long time, perhaps throughout the whole family life career. A family has to make changes in the behaviour of all members. "Moral support" given by family and friends help the patient to feel more cheerful and confident.

With respect to close relationships and illness, obligations for dealing with the day-to-day practical aspects of illness have been traditionally assigned as family responsibilities, particularly for women. There is considerable evidence that disabling chronic health problems change the relationships with family and friends (French, 1984; Lyons, 1991). Some evidences also suggest that because of illness, increased value is placed on relationships (Weinberg and Williams, 1978). Investigators have noted different effects of chronic illness on family relationships, including alteration of traditional family roles and increased psychological distress (Turk, Rudy and Flor, 1985). Dura Beck (1988) conducted a comparative study of functioning in family where mothers were experiencing chronic pain, diabetes or no illness. Data were collected on parents and children. Families with a mother who had chronic pain had poorer perceived family environments characterized by less cohesive and expressive and more controlling and conflicting relationships and higher levels of anxiety and depression as compared with other two groups.

Illness intrudes on roles and pleasures that originally constituted close relationships within family. Changes include reduced social network size, increased marital and family difficulties, reduced frequency and spontaneity in social contacts, the termination of activity based contacts and difficulties in companionate activity support and communication. One of the primary goals of a researcher is to identify which factors support and which factors constrain relationship quality and personal well-being for people with health problems.

Human beings seem to require a variety of relationships that contribute in different ways to well-being (Hirsch, 1980; Walker, MacBride and Vachon, 1977). Health challenges can threaten the stability of relationships. Reduction in shared activities, the redistribution of roles and responsibilities and changes in autonomy can strain relational bond and may cause setback to well-being. Although disabling chronic health problems are a major threat to relationships, there is also evidence that even though the most severe, life threatening illnesses, social relationships can be preserved, effectively restructured, maintained and was improved (Croog and Levine, 1977; Lyons, 1986). Relationships are sometimes reported as closer or more valued with the threat of their loss (Lyons, 1991).

A quality of life study on 1480 institutional disabled provided a disturbing profile of social isolation and inactivity among respondents (Ervionics Research Group Ltd., 1989). Kinney and Coyle (1989) conducted a study on 790 physically disabled adults. Results indicated that respondents were markedly lonely and isolated. Those who were dissatisfied with their lifestyles also tended to score low on feelings of mastery. They were usually isolated and tried to reduce stress by drinking, eating and smoking or through excessive use of tranquilizing drugs. In families the whole is greater than sum of its parts. All family members are interconnected, interdependent and exist in a fragile balance. Social support provided by family and friends contribute to life satisfaction.

Serious health problems challenge the quality and maintenance of relationships with family. At the same time such relationships play a pivotal role in coping with the constraints imposed by illness. It was found that relational difficulties are a major source of stress in individuals' attempts to cope with chronic illness and disability (Caplan, 1974; Cohen and Wills, 1985; Moos and Tsu, 1977).

The influence of personal relationships on adaptation to chronic illness has been conceptualized and studied from three orientations: (i) the social support perspective which treats personal relationships as vehicles of emotional and instrumental aid that contribute to coping with stress and to enhanced well-being (Braverman, 1983; Patrick, Morgan and Charlton, 1986), (ii) the stress or social strain orientation has been characterized by investigation of how social relationships impede well-being (Coyne and Delongis, 1986), (iii) the combined orientation viewed that relationships are contributing both positive and negative outcomes in coping with illness.

Relationships provide both support and stresses in the coping. The absence of supportive network has been linked to loneliness and negative health outcomes (Berkman, 1985; Lynch, 1977).

Gottlieb (1993) commented on the use of social support seeking as a relationship maintenance strategy. He quoted—"I began to maintain relationships with others not to alienate them by one's way of coping. The reason for drawing on relationships for coping is to shore those relationships up and the reason for coping in certain ways you or at least to believe that this is the case."

Davis-Ali, *et al.* (1994) in studying couples in which one partner had a kidney transplant have found that the nature of coping strategies is influenced by relationship's quality and social support. Patients who reported receiving more support from their significant others used more cognitive restructuring and fewer avoidant strategies (such as problem avoidance and social withdrawal) than did those with less perceived support. Family relationships provide both support and stress in the coping process. Coping and adaptation process employed by individuals, dyads and groups assist others in dealing with illness with illness stressors and for maintain valued relationships.

Coping

Different models have been proposed that conceptualize coping as an integral part of the interaction of psychological, environmental and biological factors influencing health and well-being. A person may react in many different ways while facing a difficult or stressful situation, in order to effectively adopt or adjust with the situation and to produce desirable outcome. Coping, a stabilizing factor can help individual to maintain psychosocial adaptation during stressful periods. Coping encompasses cognitive and behavioural efforts to reduce or eliminate stressful conditions and associated emotional distress (Lazarus and Folkman 1984; Moos and Schaefer, 1993). Lazarus has emphasized that coping is a process, a transaction between person and event that plays out across time and changing circumstances. Coping responses that may be effective and fruitful in one phase of the transaction may be used less or may even have different effect in other phase of transaction. Coping process is largely shaped by learning. According to Haan (1965) coping behaviour is flexible, purposive, reality oriented and differentiated.

Coping can be studied in terms of specific strategies used to handle a particular event or constraint. It can also be studied in terms of personal styles which tend to be more stable across situations. According to this line of research coping is viewed as having two major functions (i) the regulation of emotions or distress (emotion focused coping) and (ii) the management and direct confrontation with the problem that is causing distress (problem focused coping). Folkman and Lazarus (1980) have shown that both forms of coping are used in most stressful encounters and that the relative proportion of each form varies according to how the crisis is appraised (Aldwin *et al.*, 1980).

Investigators who think coping as chiefly controlled by personality may assume that coping consist of relatively spontaneous and stable behaviour patterns. Their studies are based on the exploration of individual differences in coping patterns and study coping as dependent variable. Other researchers who regard coping as mainly controlled by person's deliberate choices may assume that coping consists of deliberate mutable patterns. These researchers frame their study to understand the different kinds of coping patterns in different kinds of circumstances. They study the variations in coping patterns as independent variables. There is another possibility that an individual coping behaviour may reflect a habitual pattern that may occur without any conscious choice or response selection on the part of the person and without any apparent control by the particular environmental situation. Such a coping behaviour is considered as "coping trait", a stable characteristic of the person (Havlovic and Keenan, 1991; McCrae and Costa, 1986). From a process perspective, coping changes over time and in accordance with the situational contexts in which it occurs (Lazarus, 1993).

The early work on coping can be traced with the use of coping as a construct with psychodynamic tradition. Ego psychology has given substantial emphasis to defense mechanisms, referred to as coping devices. The research on coping makes use of many of the insights of the earlier tradition of psychodynamic defenses but with some major changes like most coping efforts are conceived of as responses to external stressors such as illness, divorce or hassles rather than responses to unconscious conflicts and the responses themselves are considered as conscious strategies. Particularly, the study of relationship between coping and health has evolved into one of the most popular topic in the coping area (Auerbach, 1989; Endler, Parker and Summerfeldt, 1993; Parker and Endler, 1992; Taylor 1990). Some of the models developed in this context are as—The first model suggests that coping strategies and behaviours have a direct effect on specific health variables (e.g. blood pressure or rate of recovery). The second model assumes that coping behaviours have indirect effect in health by creating a change in some health related behaviour (e.g. maintaining regular contact with health professionals). The third model states that coping strategies moderate or buffer the stress generated by specific health problem.

In a particular stressful situation, an unlimited number of coping strategies are available for an individual. The early coping researchers began to identify and study a number of basic coping responses (Cohen and Lazarus, 1973; Kahn *et al.* 1964; Pearlin and Scholoer, 1978; Sidle *et al.*, 1978). Two coping dimensions were identified by researchers' emotion focused coping and problem focused coping. Almost all coping measures developed in the past few decades include scales that assess these two coping dimensions (e.g. Billings and Moos, 1981; Carver, Scheier and Weintraub, 1989; Endler and Parker, 1990a, 1990b; Folkman and Lazarus, 1980, 1985; Epstein and Meier, 1989)

Other than problem focused and emotion focused coping dimensions, another basic dimension identified by early researchers is "Avoidance oriented coping." This dimension is conceptualized as an individual can react to a stressful situation by seeking out other people (social diversion) or can engage in a substitute task (distraction).

A wide variety of studies have also identified another dimension of coping response, i.e. relationship focused coping.

The coping efforts, which are serving as interpersonal regulation function has been, termed relationship focused coping (Coyne and Smith, 1991; Delongis and O'Brien, 1990). Relationship focused coping refers to those modes of coping which are oriented to managing, regulating or preserving relationship during periods of stress. To cope successfully in adverse situation may not only involve solving problems or managing emotions but may also involve maintaining and protecting social relationships. There are a number of empirical evidences which reveal the heavy cost in caring for others who are chronically ill or distressed (Stephens *et al.*, 1990).

There are a wide variety of disparate stresses such as chronic illness, natural, disaster, job loss, marital discord and the challenges of difficult examinations and even daily life hassles and so on. The individual have to face all these stressors and try to cope with them. The assessment of coping is not a simple task. A variety of techniques have been used to measure coping, including interviews, physiological measures and paper pencil inventories. Currently, several measures of coping are in widespread use as Ways of Coping Checklist (Folkman and Lazarus, 1985). Multidimensional Coping Inventory (Endler and Parker, 1990), COPE Inventory (Carver, Scheier and Weistrunb, 1989), Billings and Moos Coping Measure (Billings and Moos, 1981), Life Situation Inventory (Feifel and Strack 1989) and so on.

Aldwin and Revenson (1987) have said that we are far from describing a magic bullet coping strategy that can instantly solve problems and restore emotional equilibrium. Rather variations in what persons, contexts, events, in particular, across points of time in adaptation process success are relative. Actual coping behaviour not only is the outcome of demand or goal appraisal but also depends on demand resources and goal resources appraisal. The resources may be internal or external. External resources can be money, time, distance from professional help or the kind of social support or social network on which the patient can rely upon. Social support and relationship within family have a positive, as well as, negative relationship with adaptation to chronic disease. Manne and Zautra (1989) found that rheumatoid arthritis patients with critical, less supportive spouses are more likely to use maladaptive coping behaviours such as wishful thinking, whereas, patients with supportive spouses reported more problem focused coping.

Social support may have beneficial effects on emotional adjustment to the disease. One study found that among patients who had the most illness related disabilities, the availability of social support protected them from becoming depressed. Individuals with inadequate support were more likely to become depressed as their disabilities related to diabetes increased (Littlefield, Rodin, Murray and Craven, 1990). Social resources can bolster coping efforts by enhancing self-efficacy, as well as, providing information and guidance. Individuals who enjoyed more social resources from their family or friends relied more on approach coping such as positive reappraisal and seeking guidance and support and less on avoidance coping, especially emotional discharge (Holahan and Moos, 1987; Moos, Brenen, Fondacaro and Moos, 1990).

It has been said again and again that a focus on coping behaviours on the one hand and, social support on the other cannot be conceived of as two alternatives; rather, they are mutually supplementary perspectives (Brickman *et al.*, 1982; Fillip and Aymanns, 1987). For example—support mobilization (Eckenrode, 1983), or seeking social support (Dunkel Schetter, Folkman and Lazarus, 1987) should be expected to be successful modes of coping, their effectiveness is at the same time, dependent on and shaped by the social environment. So, not only are the individuals coping strategies themselves often highly influenced by the social context but their effectiveness is modified by the social environment as well.

Internal resources comprised of the energy or physical strength a person possesses, as well as, personality characteristics such as intelligence, trait anxiety, depression, optimism, and autonomy, ego-strength, hardiness, locus of control or self-efficacy etc. A few studies have proposed that both personality and coping are involved directly or indirectly in the production and maintenance of various kinds of maladjustment. Studies have reported a number of personality dimensions which have potential effect on coping. Lazarus (1966) described factors like affiliation and approval motives, self-esteem conformity and defensiveness. Janis (1974) reported that anxious individuals generally cope less well. Pearlin and Schooler (1978) measured self-esteem, self-denigration and mastery. Researchers have found a number of traits that explain personality (e.g. Cattell, Eber and

Tatsuoka, 1970; Eysenck and Eysenck, 1985). A newer attempt involves the five factor model of personality originally propounded by Types and Christal (1961) and recently elaborated by several researchers (e.g. McCrae, 1992 a; McCrae and Costa, 1985). Costa and McCrae (1985) suggested that the five traits of neuroticism, extraversion, openness, agreeableness and consciousness represent the core components of personality and coping styles are related to these basic five factors of personality. For example: Smith, Pope, Rhodewalt and Poulton (1989) found that trait anxiety was associated with relatively less use of problem focused coping and seeking social support and more use of wishful thinking and avoidance. Martin (1989) found that extraversion is a predictor of active coping among survivors of myocardial infraction. Grace and Schill (1986) have found that interpersonal traits, a measure of agreeableness were positively related to seeking social support.

Carver, Scheier and Pozo (1992) found that optimistic patients seem to cope in a more active, problem oriented way, whereas, pessimistic patients tend to show more passive or avoidant forms of coping. Carver *et al.* (1993) found that overt denial and behavioural disengagement were prospective predictors of greater distress among breast cancer patients and that acceptance and use of humour were prospective predictors of less distress.

Coping effectiveness implies a relationship between coping behaviours and various outcomes. Researches found that patients who use avoidant emotion focused strategies have more difficulty in adjusting to chronic disease than those who use the active problem focused strategies. For example: Research with diabetic patients showed a relationship between avoidant emotions focused coping and poor psychological adjustment (White, Richter and Fry, 1992) and on association between active problems focused coping and successful adaptation (Pollock, 1989).

Studies with patients of coronary artery heart disease (Muthny, 1992) and renal diseases and multiple sclerosis (O'Brien, 1993; Woller *et. a1*, 1992) also found that avoidant emotion focused strategies are associated with lower quality of life and/or that the use of active problem focused strategies is related to higher self-esteem, life satisfaction and or compliance with medical advice.

Sherbourne *et al.*, (1992) studied patients with hypertension, diabetes and heart diseases and found very few differences in coping behaviour between the patient groups. A general trend was found that avoidant emotion focused coping strategies are related to poor psychological adjustment and poor adherence to medical advice concerning lifestyle changes, medication and self-management, whereas, active problem focused forms of coping show a positive relationship with successful psychological and physical adjustment.

Dunkel-Schetter, Feinstein, Taylor and Falke (1992) found that cancer patients do not limit themselves to only one or two strategies. They conducted study on 668 cancer patients. Amongst them 67 per cent used at least four out of five strategies to adapt to the stressors cancer imposed on them. However, cancer patients also like most other patients suffering from chronic disease, mainly use passive emotion focused strategies, such as escape avoidance wishful thinking (de Ridder and Schreurs, 1994).

Maes and Bruggemans (1990) conducted a study on 174 coronary heart disease patients, at an average of about 5 years after the incidence. It was found that avoidance coping was negatively associated with anxiety, depression, anger, displeasure, feelings of invalidity, social inhibition and the use of medical resources, whereas, approach strategies were positively associated with these outcome variables.

Frenzel *et al.* (1988) demonstrated that up to 80 per cent of coping efforts used by diabetes patients concerned with active cognitive or behavioural strategies. Many studies had reported that it is only through active coping that diabetic patients are able to maintain their demanding regimen (Band, 1990; Grey *et al.* 1991; Spirito *et al.* 1991). In a study conducted in Indian socio-cultural context Kothari and Agarwal (1999) reported religion was the most preferred coping pattern by rural and urban patients awaiting abdominal surgery, heart surgery and cancer surgery.

The research literature on coping with chronic illness suggest that avoidant, emotion focused coping strategies are related to less efficient coping and active, problem focused coping leads to a better adjustment to chronic illness.

Quality of Life

Quality of life was earlier considered as an indicator of economic growth and upliftment of people but relatively recently it is conceptualized as an issue of psychological importance for the chronically ill. In the area of chronic illnesses earlier physicians mainly assessed the quality of life of patients. The correlations, however, between physician's ratings of patients quality of life, and that of patients own ratings or assessments by relatives, are found to be very weak. For example, in a study conducted by Jackuck, Brierley, Jackuck and Wilcox (1982) on hypertensive patients, it was found that although 100 per cent of physicians reported their patients, quality of life had improved following hypertensive medication, only half of the patients agreed, and none of the relatives did so. This suggests that quality of life is a subjective experience.

WHO has defined quality of life as "individuals' perceptions of their position in life in the context of the culture and value systems in which they live and in relation to their goals, expectations, standards and concerns." This definition also indicates that quality of life is a self-report from the individual, which is not directly related to reports or judgments of others.

Quality of life is a multidimensional concept. Growing body of researches established that quality of life is an important health outcome and must be taken into consideration in assessing the functioning of chronically ill patients. So, health related quality of life is generally assessed including such basic dimensions as physical status and functioning, psychological status, social functioning and disease or treatment related symptoms (Coons and Kaplan, 1992).

Hornquist (1989) defines quality of life as recognized need and functional satisfaction within a number of fundamental life domains with special emphasis on well-being. According to Hornquist, the quality of life concept has been operationalized to evaluate the following domains:

(i) Physical domain, which covers, overall bodily health and specific sickness impact, (ii) Psychological domain which covers satisfaction with life, well-being in general and intellectual functioning, (iii) Social domain, which covers social contact in general, as well as, specifically with sexual life and family, (iv) Behavioural/activity domains which covers capacity for self-care, work and mobility, (v) Structural domain which covers religious faith, and (vi) Material domain which covers the individuals' personal economic status.

Spilker (1990) said that one of the benefits by self-reported quality of life is that it provides information of the patient's own experiences in addition to the more traditional biomedical measures. Studies in which the patients rated the quality of life, when compared to those of the physician and nurse have shown only weak association indicating that it is the patient who is best able to express his own feelings.

Psychologists agree that the assessment of subjective experience of quality of life of patients are needed for the intervention purposes: (i) assessment of quality of life suggest the degree to which illness interferes with the quality of life of individual, (ii) assessment of quality of life can pinpoint which particular problems are likely to emerge for patients with which particular disease, (iii) assessment of quality of life is also beneficial for assessing the impact of treatment of quality of life, and (iv) a broader level information related to quality of life is useful for policy level decision-making.

Health psychologists are becoming more aware for improving the quality of life among those diagnosed with chronic illnesses, so that individuals may live their remaining years as free from pain, disability and lifestyle compromises as possible (House, Kessler and Herzog, 1990).

A study conducted by Cassileth *et al*, (1984) comprising of 758 patients each of whom had one of the six different chronic illnesses (arthritis, diabetes, cancer, renal disease, dermatologic disorder or depression) found that five of the groups did not differ significantly from one another or from the general public, but all had significantly higher scores for psychological status when compared with the sixth group, patients under treatment for depression. They state that physically ill patients remain psychologically intact and are similar to the general public in mental health.

Martins, Franca and Kimura (1996) conducted a study on 71 subjects afflicted with either high blood pressure or diabetes mellitus. The study had two objectives: to identify the significance of the quality of life of people with chronic illness and verify its interference in their quality of life. Results showed the significance of quality of life to interviewed people was related mainly to material comfort (40.9%), physical comfort (23.9%) and emotional comfort (11.2%). Chronic illness interfered with their quality of life because it had changed their physical capacity (67.6%), their work/study/home activities (64.8%) and their self-esteem (53.5%).

Hanestad (1993) studied 247 type I diabetics. The aim of the investigation was to describe how people with type I diabetes viewed their quality of life. Findings showed that over 80 per cent of patients reported the capacity for self-care, general well-being, and satisfaction with life and social contacts to be quite good or better. Forty five per cent of patients perceived their life situation to be negatively affected due to diabetes, living alone had a negative; effect on satisfaction in the physical, social and psychological life domains. In nutshell, it can be concluded that the subjective experiences of patients about their quality of life in various life domains give an insight about how to develop an intervention programme. It also ascertains whether any intervention programme had any effect or not in enhancing the perception of quality of life.

Subjective feelings and experiences and the quality of life of patients suffering from chronic illnesses are becoming recognized as important factors in the planning and evaluation of treatment strategies and intervention process. This has resulted in recognition of quality of life as an important variable along with the traditional biomedical measures (Spilker, 1990). The coping strategies, which one employs to deal with chronic illness, can also influence the quality of life of patients. Felton, Revenson and Hinrichson (1984) employed ways of coping checklist and reported that coping strategies were significantly related to quality of life even after the effects of extent of illness and demographic variables were statistically partial out.

Weisman and Worden (1976) found that when cancer patients responded immediately with social instruction, optimism and frank discussion of their condition they had relatively better mood and problem solving skills.

Coping style had also been useful in its predictions of a negative response to physical illness e.g. repression/sensitization predicted medical complication after angioplasty (Shaw *et al.*, 1986) and premorbid coping ability predicted survival after a myocardial infraction (Zikmud, Cagan and Jurkoviciva, 1983). Wagner, and Laughlin (1995) found that style of coping with cancer was related with ratings of quality of life. The more patients' suppressed competing activities to focus on their illness the worse rated their quality of life. The more religious practices were used as a method of coping; the worse were the ratings of perceived quality of life. Particularly, in the case of cancer patients to lean more towards the religion and spiritual sources to find a meaning and help to face death with dignity (Takela, 1989; Chaturvedi; 1991). Review of literature indicates that subjective feelings of patients about quality in their lives have been identified as one of the most important factors in coping with chronic diseases.

The evaluation of quality in life is increasingly dependent upon the quality and emotional judgment to various domains of life. Campbell, Converse and Rodgers (1976) suggested that personality and related issues such as self-esteem have an influence on perceived quality of life. Abbey and Andrews (1985) also suggested in their model that internal control, social support and performance resulted in increased life quality. Abbey, Abramis and Caplan (1985), Vinokur, Suhul and Caplan (1987) also reported high correlation of social support to quality of life.

Taylor, Frier, Gold and Deary (2002) examined the relationship between psychosocial variables and diabetes related outcomes in adults with newly diagnosed Type I diabetes. They found that high neuroticism diagnosis was insistently associated with poorer self-reported diabetes quality of life at 4 months and at 12 months after diagnosis. Woodruff and Convey (1990) found that reporting of lesser number of psychosomatic symptoms are related to higher evaluation of health and fitness. Psychological characteristic of optimism was found to be associated with problem focused coping on the one hand and faster recovery and higher quality of life six month after surgery, on the other hand (Scheier, Mathews and Owens, 1989). Optimism also predicted lower postpartum depression, less depression among pregnant women, less distress greater well-being and life satisfaction (Sweetman, Munz and Wheeler, 1993). Optimism has positive association with psychological and physical well-being (Vinck, Wels, Arick and Vinck, 1998).

Reviews of literature suggest that positive psychological characteristics of optimism, sense of having control, futurity, reporting lesser number of psychosomatic symptoms etc. leads to better perception of quality of life. Knowledge of the positive value of these variables is important in planning and evaluation of treatment strategies and intervention. Subjective feelings of patients quality of life has been recognized as one of the important factors in managing chronic health conditions.

Life Satisfaction

"Life satisfaction is a global assessment of a person's quality of life according to his chosen criteria" (Shin and Johnson, 1978). Satisfaction with life is a cognitive judgmental process and one of the two components of subjective well-being; the other component is the emotional or affective component (Diener and Emmons, 1984; Andrews and Withey, 1976; Veenhoven, 1984). The judgment about the domains of life by the individual is dependent upon the comparison between the existing and the standards set by the individual. Different domains of life like family, education, marriage, occupation, health and so on, are important at one time or another but life satisfaction is not the evaluation of various segments of life one by one. Veenhoven (1984) also pointed out that some people may be happy with particular domain of their life but unhappy with other or relatively satisfied with one and dissatisfied with other. Similarly, it is also possible that an individual might be satisfied with most of the domains of his life and shall be dissatisfied with life on the whole. That is why, life satisfaction is defined as a global evaluation by a person of his or her life (Deiner *et al.*, 1985). When measured in a global framework life satisfaction shows considerable stability over time (Heady and Wearing, 1989).

Most sociologists conceptualized life satisfaction as the key indicator of well-being. Life satisfaction viewed as a cognitive construct, was seen to complement happiness, one of the more affective dimensions of positive functioning. (e.g. Andrews and Makennell, 1980; Andrews and Withey, 1976; Bryant and Veroff, 1982; Campbell, Converse and Rodgers, 1976).

According to Diener *et al*, (1985) in judging about the satisfaction with their lives individuals set a standard which they perceive appropriate for circumstances of their lives to that standard. Because the standards are constructed by the individual himself, his judgment about the satisfaction with his life is based on standards set on the basis of external worldly criteria. In domain specific, evaluation of life satisfaction, such life domains as health, wealth and marital life satisfaction are chosen. Some individuals, however, may give more weight to health but not to wealth or unhappy with marital life and may feel satisfied in spite of not being wealthy. It is also possible that an individual may be satisfied with all domains of his life but may still be dissatisfied with a particular domain which he weighs as most important and this dissatisfaction with this particular domain may negatively affect overall life satisfaction. That is why, psychologists like Diener *et al.*, (1985), Heady and Wearing (1989) stated that life satisfaction when measured in a global perspective, shows stability. Life satisfaction reflects different information for different people. It may be changed depending on what is important at that particular moment. Some people may search for information about positive aspects of their lives, whereas, others might seek information about problematic areas (Diener *et al.*, In press). Similarly, people differ in the degree to which they weigh their moods and emotions while calculating life satisfaction judgments (Suh and Diener, 1999). Although life satisfaction assessed as life as-a-whole refers to stability but sufficient body of research (e.g. Pavot, Diener and Suh, 1989) suggests that judgment based on temporal is relatively more reliable and accurate. The temporality while evaluating life satisfaction focuses on the past, present and future levels of global life satisfaction. Diener and Diener (1995) also found that people in individualistic countries may base their life satisfaction judgments on the extent to which they feel high self-esteem, whereas, people in collectivistic cultures may base their judgments on the opinions of other people. Mayers and Diener (1995) said, "Satisfaction is less a matter of getting what you want than wanting what you have." For example after a period of adoption (about 3 months) even people who have experienced serious life events again report near baseline levels of well-being (Suh, Diener and Fujita, 1996).

Having effective coping mechanisms may be one of the most important predictors of well-being across the life span. Baca, George and Albertson Owens (1999) examined the relation between four types of coping strategies and life satisfaction in 224 younger adults (18-35 years) and 223 older adults (60-95 years). All participants were healthy community dwelling volunteers who were interviewed about their coping competency and their use of optimism, humour and spirituality to cope with difficult life events. Results showed no age differences on reports of health, life satisfaction and the use of optimism, humour and spirituality.

Collapsing across age, positive and statistically significant relations were observed between each of the four coping strategies and life satisfaction.

Lewinshon, Render and Seely (1991) found that life satisfaction was positively correlated with greater use of coping responses relying on cognitive self-control and negatively correlated with coping responses of maladaptive escapism and solace seeking.

Life satisfaction is a meaningful and important aspect of personality. Researches have shown that a number of psychosocial factors like optimism, locus of control, age, education, family relations etc. may have a significant and crucial role in judging global life satisfaction. According to Hanstead (1992) there are many psychosocial aspects like, having good interpersonal relations which influence individual's satisfaction with life to a greater or lesser extent?

Strack, Schwartz and Gschneidinger (1985) found that subjects who had previously been induced to think about positive aspects of their present life described themselves as happier and more satisfied with their life as a whole than subjects who had been induced to think about negative aspects. Heady and Wearing (1991) found that more satisfied people tend to be more extraverted, less neurotic and more open to feelings.

There are certain aspects of life, which are much more strongly linked to satisfaction. These are marriage and other social relationship, the condition of work and leisure activities. Campbell *et al*, (1976) in their classic study "The quality of American life" found that certain domains of satisfaction were very important for satisfaction with life as a whole. The important domains were family life and marriage. The fact is that social relationships affect all the three satisfaction components of happiness—positive affect, satisfaction and prevention of distress. Negative and positive affect are two relatively independent and additive determinants of satisfaction (e.g. Bradburn, 1969; Emmons and Deiner, 1985; Warr, 1978; Watson and Tellegon, 1985). There are some aspects of life which are not found so strongly predicting satisfaction. For example: Argyle (1987) found lack of correlation for satisfaction with education, sports facilities, crime prevention and housing.

Lewinshon, Render and Seely (1991) found that individuals with higher life satisfaction levels described themselves as having more extensive, frequent and reliable social support, as being more socially skilled and feeling more content with their relationships with others. Harlow and Cantor (1996) also found that social participation was a strong predictor of life satisfaction for retired adults. More satisfied individuals were likely to endure items indicating external locus of control for both failure and success experienced and felt they had more control over their lives and social outcomes. They were more optimistic and less pessimistic. Life satisfaction was positively correlated with self-esteem.

Numerous studies have documented that individual who perceive a supportive environment are more likely to report greater satisfaction with their lives than those who do not (e.g. Abbey, Abranis and Caplan, 1985; Vinokur, Schul and Caplan, 1987). Thus, it can be said that differences in judging think and access pleasant and unpleasant information. Cognitive dispositions like, optimism (Scheier and Carver, 1993), futurity (Pandey and Agarwal, 1998) and expectancy for control (Grob *et al.*, 1999) appear to influence satisfaction with life.

Objectives and Hypotheses

The objectives of the present investigation were decided upon with this background.

Chronic illness poses a burden on the patients, who have to live with the disease for several years and sometimes for the rest of their lives. It is, therefore, pertinent to understand the role of psychological factors, like, future orientation, optimism, personal control and symptoms reported by patients, social factors, like, family environment and behavioural factors, like, causal attribution, following treatment regimen and goals and fears of patients, in dealing with chronic illness. So, the broad aim of the present investigation is to find out the role of above-mentioned psychosocial and behavioural factors in the management of chronic illness, and attaining good quality of life and satisfaction with life.

The patients who are afflicted with a chronic disease have to face the difficulties caused by the disease in every sphere of life, whether it is workplace, home or daily routine activities. Thus, one needs coping strategies to manage the situation, hence, the aim of this investigation is also to find out those coping strategies which are effective in management of chronic illness and lead to satisfaction and good quality of life.

On the basis of above-mentioned broad aims the specific objectives of the present investigation have been outlined below:

(I) (a) Chronic illnesses pose economic problems to the patient, hamper his/her physical activities, interfere in his/her work, it bother him to change the food habits and present other kinds of challenges. And all these changes threaten his positive psychological state of mind, and use of effective coping strategies. So, the first aim of the present investigation is to examine the role of psychological factors, like, future orientation, optimism, personal control and symptom reporting in using effective coping strategies to overcome stressors.

(b) Chronic illnesses not only affect the psychological state of the patient but also interfere in the functioning of family. A large number of studies suggest that the kind of social support, social network and family bonding etc. which is available increases or decreases the likelihood of successfully overcoming the stressors. It is, thus, understood that the use of effective coping strategies is influenced by social factor. The second aim of this research work is also to delineate social factor, like, family environment as perceived by the victim himself which influences the use of various coping strategies.

(2) A number of studies have revealed that satisfaction with life and quality of life have a number of psychosocial correlates, such as age, income, marital status and psychological variables, like, future orientation, optimism, self-efficacy, self-mastery and personality related factors like, sense of personal control and social factors like, family environment. So, the third aim of the present investigation is to examine the predictive value of psychosocial factors in achieving greater satisfaction and better quality of life in patients of chronic diseases, as well as, respondents of non-patient group.

(3) Effective coping strategies may lead to better perception of quality of life and satisfaction with life and ineffective coping strategies may lead to poor perception of quality of life and lesser satisfaction with life. So, the forth aim of the present investigation is to explore and pinpoint those coping strategies which predict greater satisfaction with life and a better quality in life.

(4) It has been observed by many researchers that behavioural factors, like, the causes attributed by individuals for their

awesome conditions, the goals set by persons for themselves and the kind of fears they possess, may influence the types of coping strategies used by them and also their perception of quality of life and satisfaction with life. So, the next aim of this investigation is to find out the role of these behavioural factors in perception of quality of life and satisfaction with life.

On the basis of above-mentioned objectives of the present investigation following hypotheses have been framed:

(1) It is hypothesized that psychological factors, like, future orientation, optimism and personal control will positively predict the use of active and adaptive coping strategies and symptoms reported will negatively predict the use of active and adaptive coping strategies.

(2) It is hypothesized that psychological factors, like, future orientation, optimism and personal control will negatively predict the use of maladaptive coping strategies and symptoms reported will positively predict the use of maladaptive coping strategies.

(3) It is hypothesized that social factors, like, relationship in family, opportunities for personal growth in family and system maintenance in family, will positively predict the use of active and adaptive coping strategies and negatively predict the use of maladaptive coping strategies.

(4) It is hypothesized that psychological factors, like, future orientation, optimism and personal control will positively predict better perception of quality of life and satisfaction with life and symptoms reporting will negatively predict better perception of quality of life and satisfaction with life.

(5) It is hypothesized that social factors, like, relationship in family, opportunities for personal growth in family and system maintenance in family will positively predict the better perception of quality of life and satisfaction with life.

(6) It is hypothesized that the use of active and adaptive coping strategies will lead to better perception of quality of life and satisfaction with life.

(7) It is hypothesized that the use of maladaptive coping strategies will lead to poor, perception of quality of life and satisfaction with life.
(8) It is hypothesized that the differences in behavioural factors like the causes attributed by the person, the goals set by him/her or the fears possessed by him/her will lead to difference in perception of quality of life and satisfaction with life.

Method

Sample

The sample consisted of a total of 235 participants. Amongst them 180 (90 males and 90 females) were patients suffering from any of the three chronic illnesses, *viz*. Diabetes, cardiovascular problems and cancer and 55 participants (30 males and 25 females) were non-patient healthy group of participants, who did not have any chronic or acute illness. They served as control group. The criteria used to select individuals as participants was as follows:

For Chronically Ill Patient Groups

(i) Those participants who were suffering from type II diabetes for not less than two years, were requested to participate in this study,
(ii) Those participants, who were suffering from any of the two cardiovascular problems, namely, angina or Myocardial Infraction (MI) for not less than two years, were enrolled to participate in this investigation.
(iii) Only those respondents who were suffering from either oral or breast cancer which was diagnosed at least 4 months ago and were on 2nd or 3rd stage of cancer and according to their doctor the prognosis of their survival was good were selected for participating in the present investigation.

Non-Patient Healthy Group

The non-patient healthy group comprised the participants, who had no chronic or acute illness at present or in the past. They only suffered from minor health problems, like, fever or stomach pain. The data was collected on patients in the Out Patient Department (OPD) of BRD Medical College, Gorakhpur, Hanuman Prasad Poddar Cancer Hospital, Gorakhpur and clinics of private doctors. Data was collected from non-patient healthy group of participants at their residences.

Amongst cancer patients all of the 15 male cancer patients were suffering from oral cancer diagnosed as early as four months ago and their disease was either in 2nd or in 3rd stage. The chief cause of their disease as told by patients themselves was chewing tobacco and *gutkha* or *panmasala*. The prognosis of their cancer to be treated and cured was very good according to their doctor. All of them were hospitalized for radiotherapy or chemotherapy sessions for not less than 15 days.

Table 1: Demographic Characteristics of Participants

Groups	*Diabetic Patients*	*Cancer Patients*	*Cardio-vascular Patients*	*Patient with both Diabetes, Heart Disease*	*Non-patient Healthy Group*
Male	30	15	27	18	30
Female	25	20	28	17	25
Total number	55	35	55	35	55
Average Age (in yrs)	52.40	49.17	51.30	53.94	48.85
Education (in yrs)	14.80	15.05	14.25	14.48	15.23
Annual Income	1,56,528.60	1,34,745.5	1,25,563.60	1,35,800.00	1,74,156.41

Amongst the female cancer patients all 20 patients were suffering from breast cancer. They were hospitalized for surgery, i.e. removal of cancerous part of the breast. Their surgery was going to take place within a week. They were contacted before surgery. Their doctor told that after surgery the chances of recovery and removal of cancer was good.

All the diabetic and heart patients gone through acute episode of complications related with their disease nearly one month ago, when they contacted to participate in the study. According to their doctors, they were doing well at the time of data collection.

Materials

Data Sheet for Personal Information: Two types of personal data sheets were prepared, one for chronically ill patients and one for non-patient healthy group of participants. Both of the data sheets included name, age, sex, occupation, and education, and marital status, no. of children, address for further correspondence and telephone no. of the participants.

In the personal data sheet of the chronically ill patients some other information about their disease were sought. Participants were assured that their responses would be kept secret and used only for research purposes. Consent of participants to participate in the study was procured.

An Interview schedule was prepared for chronically ill group of participants. In this interview schedule information related with chronic disease and patients' perception about disease had been asked. The information sought out in this interview schedule are given below—

1. Name of the chronic disease.
2. How long have you been afflicted with the disease?
3. Did anyone in your family suffer from disease earlier?
4. How are you related to him/her?
5. Do you follow the treatment regimen fully or not?
6. How much time will it take to reach the nearest doctor in case of emergency?
7. What was the first reaction of the family members, when you were diagnosed to have chronic disease?
8. What are the causes with you think are responsible for your disease?
9. Do you perceive that this long-term illness has resulted in anything positive? Like what.
10. List your goals and aspirations.
11. List your fears.

This information had been taken from chronically ill patients, groups of participants only. The informations given by chronically ill participants were analyzed and interpreted.

Measures

Future Orientation (FO) Story Writing Technique

Future orientation was measured by using story writing technique which is a variation of the technique used by Meade (1972). This technique was successfully adopted and used by Agrawal and Tripathi (1979) and Agrawal (1980). Four cue sentences were presented to subjects, who were asked to write a small description of what was happening or will happen, on the basis of the event described in the cue sentence. All the cue sentences were in present tense. The respondent was given eight minutes of time to write each story. Proportion of the future events, taking place after the event in the cue sentence in every story was calculated and added. The formula for calculation of proportion for future events is—

Proportion for future events = Total Future Events/Total Events

The proportion was converted into arcsinev $\sqrt{x}$ to get the future orientation score.

Data on validity of this story writing technique has accumulated over a period of last 20 years. Agarwal and Srivastava (1981), Agarwal, Srivastava and Tiwari (1984), Agrawal (2003) have found that people with reflective cognitive style as opposed to impulsive fast accurate and slow inaccurate differed significantly in their future orientation scores. Those who had reflective cognitive style were significantly more future oriented. It has been noted that those persons who have high dispositional future orientation are prone to view a task as an open task (Agarwal, 1993). This tendency leads dispositional future orientation to facilitate temporal coding. This data is congruent with theoretical formulation that a reflective cognitive style takes into account several alternatives as the correct alternative. This characteristic promotes the tendency to think future alternatives also, hence, the relationship between the two. Dispositional future orientation mediated the perception of the utility of a material in the future, to affect its temporal coding (Agarwal and Tiwari, 1988). High future oriented persons were developed favourable attitude towards those persons whose names were associated with future oriented cue statements (Tiwari and Agarwal, 1989). This tendency was significantly more evident in high as compared to low future oriented subjects. This showed the role of future orientation for formation of other unrelated attitudes. Agarwal and Pandey (1998) noted that since, future oriented patients are able to visualize hurdles is their path of achieving their goals they also think and plan about ways and means of overcoming these hurdles and maintain an optimistic outlook in spite of health problems. It was also noted by Agarwal and Tripathi (2003) that if the mothers of chronically ill children had future expectations about their children and had beliefs that health problems could be overcome in future by following present regimens, their children displayed better academic behaviour. Furthermore, mother's future expectations significantly predicted academic behaviour of children with chronic illness, normal healthy and total group of children.

The plethora of studies provides ample evidence about the theoretical soundness of the concept of future orientation and the validity of story writing technique of measurement of future orientation.

Life Orientation Test (LOT)

Dispositional optimism was measured by using the Life Orientation Test (LOT) developed by Scheier and Carver (1985). LOT is self-report measure of nine items. In addition to these there are four filler items. LOT assesses individual differences in global optimism defined in terms of generalized expectancies for positive versus negative outcomes. The scale has an internal reliability (Cronbach alpha) of 0.76 and test-retest reliability (over a 4 week interval) of 0.79 (Scheier and Carver, 1985). The retest reliability of the Hindi version of the LOT was found to be high, i.e. ($r = 0.70$) by present researcher. Participants were asked to indicate degree of agreement with each item of the scale on a five point scale ranging from (1) strongly disagree, (2) disagree, (3) neutral, (4) agree, (5) strongly agree. Five items of LOT are scored in positive (item nos. 1, 4, 5, 11, 13) and four in negative direction (item nos. 3, 8, 9, 12). After reversing the scoring for the negatively worded items, item scores were totalled. Scores of the filler items were not included in the total sum of score on dispositional optimism items. One can get a maximum of 45 and minimum of 9 score on this test. The high score represents greater optimism. Examples of the positively worded and negatively worded items are, respectively, "In uncertain times, I expect the best" and "I hardly ever expect things to go my way".

Personal Control Scale

This questionnaire of personal control was developed by M. Agarwal, A.K. Dalal, D.K. Agarwal and R.K. Agrawal (1994). This measure referred to patients' perceived controllability over their lives in general. This scale consists of 8 items dealing with patients' perception of personal control over different domains of life, like, family happiness and peace, occupational success, own health, mental peace, future events, financial security, fulfilment of goals, future peace and happiness. The items are rated on a five point scale ranging from (1) no control to (5) total control. The maximum score on this scale is 40 and the minimum is 8. The higher score denotes the greater degree of personal control. The coefficient alpha for this scale was found 0.78.

PGI Health Questionnaire N-l

This checklist was developed by Verma, Wig and Pershad (1985). This consists of a total of 38 items divided into two areas, A and B. Items in the area A were related to physical distress and items in the area B were related to psychological distress. There were 16 items in area A (Physical distress) and 22 items in area B (Psychological distress.) The psychometric properties of the test were found to be significantly high. Reliability of the test using retest and split half methods was found to be significantly high (0.80 and 0.86 respectively). For the scores the respondents had to put a tick (√) against questions he/she agreed with. The number of ticks on sections A and B indicate the respective scores, which can then be added up to give a total score. The high score on this questionnaire need not always indicate neurosis but it shows a propensity to develop neurotic symptoms under stress. The examples of one item from each section are as—"I frequently suffer from headaches" (Area A physical distress) "I get disturbed meeting new persons or going to new place." (Area B, Psychological distress)

Family Environment Scale

This scale was developed by Bhatia and Chadha (1993). The scale is based on the family environment scale developed by Moos (1974). This scale is completely an indigenous tool for measuring the type of relationship within family, opportunities for personal growth in family and value of organization and control within family. This scale consists of three dimensions. These are—**Relationship dimension,** Expressiveness, Conflict and Acceptance and caring. **Personal growth dimension**—(i) Independence, Active Recreational Orientation. **System Maintenance dimension**—Organization and Control. There are 69 items in this scale. Each item is scored on a five-point scale. Score of (5) is awarded for strongly agree and a score of (1) for strongly disagree. A number of items are negatively worded, so scoring for them was reversed. The reliability of the scale was found to be 0.95.

Coping Operation Preference Enquiry (COPE)

Dispositional coping style was assessed by Coping Operation Preference Enquiry (COPE) developed by Carver, Scheier and Weintraub (1989). COPE consists of sixty items which were divided into fifteen sub-scales having four items in each scale. Each scale emphasized a particular aspect of coping. This inventory measures a wide range of potential responses to stressors and also distinguishes each coping quality. Different stressful events bring out somewhat different patterns of responses. Respondents were asked to indicate how would they react to stressors they encountered them? They were asked to give, their responses on a 4 point scale as—(1) I usually don't do this at all, (2) I usually do this a little bit, (3) I usually do this a medium amount, (4) I usually do this a lot.

The COPE items have been factor analyzed and have moderately high test-retest reliability (Carver *et al.*, 1989). Dispositional coping styles measured through this scale and the example of each coping style is given below—Positive Reinterpretation and Growth—"I try to grow as a person as a result of the experience." Active coping—"I concentrate my efforts on doing something about it." Planning—"I make a plan of action." Seeking of Social Support for Emotional Reasons—"I discuss my feeling with someone." Seeking of Social Support for Instrumental Reasons—"I try to get advice from someone about what to do." Suppression of Competing Activities—"I put aside other activities in order to concentrate on this." Religion—"I put my trust in God." Acceptance—"I get used to the idea that it happened". Mental Disengagement—"I daydream about things other than this." Focus on and Venting of emotions—"I get upset and let my emotions out." Behavioural Disengagement—"I admit to myself that I can't [deal with and quit trying." Denial—"I refuse to believe that it has happened." Restraint coping—"I force myself to wait for the right time to do something." Alcohol/Drug use—"I use alcohol or drugs to make myself feel better." *Humour*—"I laugh about the situation."

WHO Quality of Life Scale (WHOQOL)

In order to assess the quality of life in health care settings in India, this questionnaire was developed by a team of researchers of World Health Organization (WHO), namely Saxena, Chandirmani and Bhargava (1998). The scale consists of 100 items related to four domains, namely, Physical Health, Psychological Health, Social Relationships and Environment. Each domain has a number of facets and in each facet there are four items. The facets related to each domain are:

Physical Health: Activities of daily living, Dependence on medicinal substances and medical aid, Energy and fatigue, Mobility, Pain and Discomfort, Sleep and rest, Work Capacity.

Psychological Health: Body image and Appearance, Negative Feelings, Positive Feelings, Self-Esteem, Spirituality/Religion/Personal Belief, Thinking, learning, memory, concentration.

Social Relationships: Personal Relation, Social Support, and Sexual Activity.

Environmental Health: Financial Resources, Freedom, Physical Safety and Security, Health and Social Care Accessibility and Quality, Home Environment, Opportunities for acquiring new information and skills, Participation in and opportunities for recreational/leisure activities, Physical environment pollution/noise/traffic/climate, Transport.

The Cronbach alpha for this scale was moderately high for most of the facets. All facets were significantly correlated with their respective domains. All items of WHOQOL-100 distinguished significantly between the "diseased" and "healthy". The scoring was done on a five point scale. Some of the items in the scale are positively worded and some are negatively. So the scoring for positively worded item was (5) for strongly satisfied to (1) for strongly dissatisfied and *vice versa* for negatively worded items. The retest reliability of Hindi version of this scale was 0.67 and split-half reliability was 0.71 by the present researcher.

Temporal Satisfaction With Life Scale (TSWLS)

To assess the respondent's past, present and future life satisfaction, the Temporal Satisfaction With Life Scale (TSWLS) was used. Pavot, Diener and Suh (1998) developed this scale. This scale consists of fifteen items. Amongst them five items were related to past satisfaction, five to present satisfaction and five to future satisfaction. All the items of TSWLS were keyed in a positive direction. The items were scored on a seven-point scale ranged from (1) strongly disagree to (7) strongly agree. All the items were positively keyed; therefore, scoring the TSWLS involves a summation of the 15 items. Scores on the scale could range from 15 to 105. Each sub-scale would have a response range of 5 to 35 and means on each of the sub-scale would be statistically comparable. The alpha reliability of the test was found to be 0.92 and retest reliability (a 4-week interval) was 0.83 (Pavot, Diener and Suh, 1998). The present researcher has translated this scale into Hindi language. This Hindi version of the scale was significantly and positively correlated (r = 0.79) with that of original English version. The retest reliability of Hindi version, after an interval of 8 weeks was 0.77. This scale was also correlated with short version of satisfaction with life scale and a coefficient of correlation of 0.74 was found. Examples of the past, present and future sub-scales of the TSWLS are—"I am satisfied with my life in the past" (Past). "I am satisfied with my current life" (Present) "I will be satisfied with my life in the future" (Future).

Procedure

The main purpose of this study was to find out the role of some psychosocial variables in living with chronic diseases in general, and coping with the troublesome treatment regimen in particular and also find out the type of coping strategies used by persons afflicted with anyone of the chronic diseases, namely, diabetes, cancer or cardiovascular problems. In order to fulfil the aim of the study the process of data collection was started with contacting each patients afflicted with above-mentioned chronic illnesses in hospitals. The patients were selected on the basis of criteria outlined earlier.

Data was collected in two sessions. In the first session the scales of optimism, family environment, personal control, temporal satisfaction with life and coping were given and in the second session the future orientation story writing technique, quality of life scale and PGI health questionnaire are given. All the cancer patients were contacted at the Hanuman Prasad Podder Cancer Hospital, Gita Vatika, Gorakhpur. The male cancer patients suffering from oral cancer were being treated with radiotherapy and chemotherapy. All of them were hospitalized for at least 7 to 15 days. The purpose of the study was disclosed to them and they were requested to participate in the study. After their consent the instructions were read to the patients and they were asked whether they were able to understand the instructions.

For those respondents who expressed their inability to fill-up the questionnaires the researcher herself filled up the questionnaire. The data was collected on women cancer patients in the same manner. The women cancer patients, who were afflicted with breast cancer, were hospitalized for surgery.

In the next phase of the study the data was collected on patients afflicted with either type II diabetes or heart problems i.e., angina or myocardial infraction. The patients suffering from these diseases were contacted at the Out Patient Department of B.R.D. Medical College, Gorakhpur and a number of private clinics and at their homes. Data collection was lengthy hence, in the first session these patients were contacted in the OPDs and into the second session at their homes. Most of the heart and diabetic patients fulfilled their questionnaires by themselves, but their answers were probed. While collecting the data on diabetic and heart patients, the researcher came across a number of patients who were suffering from both diabetes and heart problems, hence, a separate category of these patients was formed.

In order to collect the information from non-patient healthy group of respondents the researcher contacted a number of persons at their homes. Those who fulfilled the criteria to be a participant in the study were enrolled in the study. The purpose of the study was disclosed to them and they were requested to participate in the investigation. The data was collected on the same questionnaires as described earlier from these participants. The only difference was that the personal data sheet used for patient group has questions related to their disease was not given to them. For non-patient group of participants only their name, age, sex, etc. had been asked. The entire non-patients healthy group of participants filled up their protocol by themselves. For the non-patient healthy group of participants the data collection procedure was also completed in two sessions. In this way a total of 180 chronically ill patients and 55 healthy individuals were contacted individually in two sessions.

After the completion of data collection process, each protocol has been rechecked and if there had been anything left or missing, the researcher personally contacted the participants again. Sometimes, a person filled the protocol in the first session, but due to some reason or the other was not available in the second session. Such protocols were dropped in the analysis. Twenty protocols, 15 from chronically ill group and 5 from healthy group had to be abandoned. The measuring tools were scored in their respective ways according to manual instructions.

Results

The "biopsychosocial" model of health implies that any health or illness outcome is a consequence of the interplay of biological, psychological and social factors (Engel, 1977; Schwartz, 1982). The fundamental point of this model is that health and illness are caused by multiple factors and produce multiple effects. The psychosocial factors of future orientation, optimism, personal control and symptoms reported were psychological factors and family environment was a social factor. Besides these a number of demographic variables like, age, income and education were matched because various studies (Campbell, Converse and Rodgers 1976) have shown that sometimes these demographic variables may interact with the contribution of psychological and social factors in coping with stress and perception of quality of life and satisfaction with life. The results were analyzed and presented in five sections.

SECTION-A

Descriptive statistics has been presented in this section.

Frequency and Percentages of Some Treatment and Disease Related Response

Table 2 shows frequency of history of the chronic diseases in the families of patients and also how much the patients were following the treatment regimen. This table revealed that none of cancer patient had a history of any type of cancer in their families and also the cancer patients were following the treatment regimen fully but not the other three groups of patients.

Table 2: Treatment and Disease Related Responses

Groups	*Cancer Patients*	*Diabetic Patients*	*Heart Patients*	*Patients with both D&H*
Family History of Disease				
– Present	0	38	27	25
– Absent	35	17	28	10
Following Treatment Regimen				
– Fully	100%	36.36%	47.27%	80%
– Partially	–	63.63%	52.72%	20%

Means and Standard Deviations of Psychosocial Variables

Table 3 presents the means and standard deviations of psychological variables (future orientation, optimism, personal control and symptoms reported by participants) and social variables (relationship in family, opportunities for personal growth in family, and system maintenance in family) for chronically ill, healthy and pooled group of participants.

SECTION-B

Differential use of various **coping strategies** by participants groups were analyzed and been presented in this section "B".

Global Coping Strategies as used by Different Groups: The means and standard deviations of coping strategies used by the patient groups of participants suffering from cancer, diabetes and heart problems, and healthy group of participants to cope up with stress was presented in Table 4. This also presents the mean scores of coping strategies as used by four groups of participants suffering from chronic diseases.

Coping Strategies and Psychosocial Variables

The coefficient of correlation of components of global coping strategies and different psychological and social variables has been presented in Tables 5 and 6 respectively. A close look at the table

Table 3: Means and Standard Deviations of Psychosocial Variables

Psychosocial Variables	*Cancer Patients*	*Diabetic Patients*	*Heart Patients*	*Patients with both D&H*	*Healthy Group*
Future Orientation	.94 (.22)	.97 (.21)	.97 (.26)	.99 (.11)	1.09 (.31)
Optimism	23.51 (6.19)	27.32 (4.50)	27.25 (4.33)	26.42 (3.99)	28.70 (4.17)
Personal Control	14.91 (5.93)	18.80 (7.02)	19.50 (6.82)	21.48 (6.45)	28.60 (6.33)
Physical symptoms reported	8.65 (3.14)	6.12 (2.51)	5.18 (3.67)	9.60 (2.87)	3.01 (2.48)
Psychological symptoms reported	7.94 (3.14)	10.10 (2.51)	9.60 (3.67)	8.02 (2.87)	3.74 (2.48)
Total symptoms reported	16.60 (4.13)	16.23 (4.32)	15.41 (4.87)	17.62 (6.10)	6.76 (4.06)
Relationship in family	160.91 (22.85)	161.45 (15.07)	170.14 (13.13)	152.08 (9.14)	173.60 (17.86)
Personal growth in family	52.20 (6.94)	53.65 (6.81)	58.21 (7.22)	50.28 (9.45)	61.78 (6.25)
System maintenance in family	20.40 (5.71)	20.36 (3.21)	22.67 (3.50)	20.54 (2.88)	25.70 (2.19)

Note: Standard Deviations in parentheses.

Table 4: Means and Standard Deviations of Global Coping Strategies

Coping Strategies	*Cancer Patients*	*Diabetic Patients*	*Heart Patients*	*Patients with both D&H*	*Healthy Group*
Combined Active Coping	58.57 (11.71)	60.89 (5.71)	60.76 (6.63)	59.65 (9.43)	65.92 (11.58)
Adaptive Coping	37.65 (6.62)	35.25 (4.83)	33.38 (4.41)	31.74 (2.75)	32.87 (5.66)
Maladaptive Coping	41.42 (5.72)	39.69 (4.96)	39.29 (4.56)	39.88 (4.41)	33.54 (4.92)
Acceptance Coping	11.48 (2.76)	11.45 (2.78)	11.18 (1.87)	12.08 (2.21)	10.69 (2.49)
Humour Coping	8.28 (2.60)	7.36 (3.06)	7.96 (2.68)	6.88 (1.71)	8.41 (2.49)

Note: Standard Deviations in parentheses.

Table 5: Coefficient of Correlation of Components of Global Coping Strategies and Psychological Variables

Coping Strategies	*Groups*	*Optimism*	*Future Orientation*	*Perceived Control*	*Physical Symptoms Reported*	*Psychological Symptoms Reported*	*Total Symptoms Reported*
Positive Reinterpretation	CIG	.21**	.26**	.27**	.13	.07	.13
	HG	.12	-.13	.08	.03	.28**	.26
Planning	CIG	.19**	.28**	.39**	-.22**	.03	-.12
	HG	-.14	.20	.05	.07	.02	-.27**
Active Coping	CIG	.22**	.24**	.41**	-.14	-.12	-.17*
	HG	-.05	-.05	.16	.05	-.09	-.06
Restraint Coping	CIG	.29**	.29**	.20**	-.08	-.07	-.10
	HG	.32*	.12	.22	-.12	-.14	-.18
Suppression of Competing Activities	CIG	.16**	.31**	.24**	.06	.09	.04
	HG	.02	-.03	.13	-.03	-.07	-.01
Combined Active Coping	CIG	.34**	.43**	.46**	-.15*	-.12	-.18*
	HG	.12	.01	.24	.009	.01	.02
Religion	CIG	-.18*	-.15*	-.27**	.10	.13	.15*
	HG	.05	-.27*	.003	.03	.14	.13
Instrumental Social Support	CIG	.15*	.16*	.05	-.06	.09	.03
	HG	-.02	.04	.01	.17	.22	.27
Emotional Social Support	CIG	-.08	.03	-.04	.08	.04	.08
	HG	-.18	-.18	-.26	.21	.02	.12
Adaptive Coping	CIG	-.03	.04	-.09	.05	.12	.11
	HG	-.06	-.18	-.10	.18	.17	.23
Venting off emotions	CIG	-33**	-.11	-.14	.21**	.15**	.24**
	HG	-36**	-.34**	-.39**	.16	.36**	.39**
Mental disengagement	CIG	-.14	.25**	-.38**	-.13	-.02	.21
	HG	.02	-.23	.22	.04	.21	.26**
Behavioural disengagement	CIG	-.17*	.15	-.02	.13	-.09	.03
	HG	-.06	.02	-.01	.11	.28**	.29**
Denial	CIG	.05	.05	.21**	.01	-.10	-.06
	HG	.14	.18	.16	-.11	.14	-.02
Maladaptive Coping	CIG	-.30**	-.11	-.18**	.12	-.03	.05
	HG	-.16	-.19	-.13	.20	.45**	.44**
Acceptance Coping	CIG	.04	.08	.04	.07	-.07	.01
	HG	.16	-.14	.17	-.17	-.01	-.19
Humour Coping	CIG	-.02	.04	.09	-.15*	-.17	-.15*
	HG	.66**	.06	.12	-.25	-.01	-.13

Note: P<.01**, P<.05* CIG = Chronically Ill Group
HG = Healthy Group

Table 6: Coefficient of Correlation of Components of Global Coping Strategies and Social Variables

Coping Strategies	*Groups*	*Relationship in Family*	*Personal Growth in Family*	*System Maintenance in Family*
Positive Reinterpretation	CIG	.18**	.04	.11
	HG	-.17	-.01	-.13
Planning	CIG	.09	.09	.10
	HG	-.25	-.01	.13
Active Coping	CIG	.33**	.21*	.21**
	HG	.04	-.13	.11
Restraint Coping	CIG	.25**	-.05	.35**
	HG	.05	-.18	-.22
Suppression of Competing Activities	CIG	-.08	-.01	.15*
	HG	-.04	.15	.02
Combined Active Coping	CIG	.30**	.05	.30**
	HG	-.10	-.10	-.04
Religion	CIG	.06	-.02	.03
	HG	-.04	-.11	.06
Instrumental Social Support	CIG	.23**	-.09	.17
	HG	.10	-.13	-.02
Emotional Social Support	CIG	.07	-.18*	.03
	HG	.19	.01	.10
Adaptive Coping	CIG	.18*	-.14	.12
	HG	.11	-.11	.06
Venting off emotions	CIG	-.11	-.02	-.09
	HG	.08	.02	.07
Mental disengagement	CIG	.13	.09	.02
	HG	.01	.08	-.02
Behavioural disengagement	CIG	-.23**	-.18*	-.13
	HG	-.15	.01	-.01
Denial	CIG	.07	.15*	.13
	HG	.05	-.14	-.05
Maladaptive Coping	CIG	-.10	-.01	.00
	HG	-.09	-.21**	-.27**
Acceptance Coping	CIG	-.13	-.22	.07
	HG	-.03	-.13*	-.17**
Humour Coping	CIG	.03	-.04	.11
	HG	.02	-.11	-.03

Note: P<.01**, P<.05*. CIG = Chronically Ill Group
HG = Healthy Group

showed the significant correlations amongst the components of global coping strategies and psychosocial variables in Chronically Ill Group (CIG) and Healthy Group (HG).

Psychosocial Variables as Predictors of Coping Strategies

To investigate the joint and independent contribution of psychosocial variables, namely, optimism, future orientation, personal control, symptoms reported and family environment, in coping with the rigorous treatment regimen and thorough management of chronic illness the regression analysis was done. In the regression analysis, the psychological variables used as predictors were—optimism, future orientation, personal control and symptoms reported (physical symptoms, psychological symptoms and total symptoms and the social variable, family environment (relationship in family, opportunities for personal growth in family and system maintenance in family). The type of coping strategies as used by both chronically ill and healthy group of participants were treated as criterion variables. The regression analysis was computed for all the sixteen coping strategies (as described in method section) Amongst, these coping strategies the scores of some similar kind of coping strategies were chunked together to examine their joint contribution. These chunks were (i) Combined Active coping strategies (positive reinterpretation + active coping + planning + restraint coping + suppression of competing activities), (ii) Adaptive coping strategies (religion + instrumental social support + emotional social support), (iii) Maladaptive coping strategies of emotions + mental disengagement + behavioural disengagement + denial). The results of the Stepwise Multiple Regression Analyses (SMRA) were as follows—

Combined Active Coping Strategies as Predicted by Psychosocial Variables: In chronically ill group of participants results of the SMRA identified a set of three best predictors, namely, personal control, optimism and future orientation [$F(1,179) = 22.45$, $P<.000$] in predicting combined active coping strategies to cope with stress. These three variables together explained 27.7 per cent of total variance in the criterion variable. Personal control was found the best among all three predictors which was explaining 21.2 per cent of variance in the criterion variable independently, followed by optimism which accounted for 3.5 per cent of variance, then come future orientation which was found responsible for 3 per cent of variance in the criterion variable (Table 7). However, examination of the beta values and R^2 change suggest that all these predictors were contributing positively in the criterion variable.

Table 7: Psychosocial Variables as Predictors of Combined Active Coping Strategies in Chronically Ill Group

Criterion = Combined Active Coping					
Predictors	**R**	**R^2**	**R^2 Change**	**Beta**	**t**
Psychological Variables					
Perceived Control	.46	.21	.21	.26	3.12**
Optimism	.49	.25	.035	.18	2.17**
Future Orientation	.52	.28	.03	.22	2.69**
Social Variables					
Relationship in family	.30	.09	.092	.22	2.87**
System maintenance in family	.36	.13	.039	.21	2.82**

Note: P < .01**

Table 7 also shows that in chronically ill group of participants combined active coping strategies was also predicted by social variables, relationship in family and system maintenance in family [F(1,179) = 13.40, P<.000]. These two variables together positively explained 13.1 per cent of total variance in the criterion variable. Relationship in family was found best predictor which was explaining 9.2 per cent of variance in the criterion variable independently, followed by, system maintenance in family which accounted for 3.9 per cent of variance in the criterion variable. In healthy group of participants none of the psychosocial variable was significantly contributing in the prediction of using combined active coping strategies.

How psychological variables predicted the use of global coping strategies in different patient groups was shown in Tables 8 and 9. Table 8 shows that in cancer patient group of participants two psychological variables, namely, personal control and future orientation. [F (1, 34) = 15.37, P<.000] had emerged as best predictors. These two variables jointly and positively explained 48.9 per cent variance in the criterion variable. Personal control was the best predictor which explained 41.6 per cent variance in the criterion variable independently, followed by, future orientation which accounted for 7.3 per cent variance. Table 9 shows that in cancer patient group of participants social variable, system maintenance in family [F (1, 34) = 14.64, P<.01] also accounted for 30.7 per cent variance in the criterion variable, combined active coping strategies.

In the participants of diabetes group also personal control [F (1,54) = 15.07, P<.000] (Table 8) predicted combined active strategies. Personal control positively explained 20.7 per cent variance in the criterion variable. In this group none of the social variables predicted combined active coping strategies.

In the heart patient group of participants a set of two psychological variables, namely, personal control and total symptoms reported [F (1, 54) = 10.99, P<.002] predicted combined active coping strategies. Personal control was the best predictor which explained 17.2 per cent variance independently, followed by total symptoms reported which accounted for 7 per cent variance in the criterion variables. Beta values indicated that personal control had a positive contribution whereas, total symptoms reported had negative contribution in the criterion variable (Table 8). Table 9 shows that in heart patient group of participants combined active coping strategies were also predicted social variable, relationship in family [F(1,54) = 4.03, P<.05] which accounted for 26.6 per cent variance in the criterion variable. It had positive contribution.

In the group of participants suffering from both diabetes and heart problems combined active coping strategies was predicted by future orientation [F (1, 34) = 19.378, P<.000]. Future orientation positively explained 37 per cent variance in the criterion variable (Table 8). In this group of participants combined active coping strategies was also predicted by social variables personal growth in family [F (1, 54) = 4.67, P<.03] which positively accounted for 12.4 per cent variance in the criterion variable (Table 9). Relationship in family positively explained 3.5 per cent variance in the criterion variable independently, and then come opportunities for personal growth in family which negatively accounted for 6 per cent variance in the criterion variable. In cancer patients group of participants adaptive coping strategies were predicted by a set of two psychological variables, optimism and psychological symptoms reported [F (1, 34) = 8.78, P<.000] (Table 8). These two variables together explained 35.4 per cent variance in the criterion variable independently, followed by psychological symptoms reported, which also positively accounted for 14.7 per cent variance in the criterion variable. In the group of patients suffering from diabetes and heart problems, psychological variable, physical symptoms reported [F (1, 34) = 7.49, P<.01] significantly and positively predicted adaptive coping strategies. Physical symptoms reported explained 18.5 per cent variance in the criterion variable (Table 8). In this group of participants two social variables, relationship in family and system maintenance in family [F (1, 34) = 15.22, P<.01] predicted adaptive coping strategies. These two

Table 8: Global Coping Strategies as Predicted by Psychological Variables in Patient and Healthy Groups

Criterion = Combined Active Coping Strategies						
Group	**Predictor**	**R**	**R^2**	**R^2 Change**	**Beta**	**t**
Cancer Patients	Perceived Control Future Orientation	.65 .70	.41 .49	.41 .073	.42 .35	2.53** 2.14**
Diabetic Patients	Perceived control	.47	.22	.20	.47	3.88**
Heart Patients	Perceived Control Symptoms Reported	.41 .49	.17 .24	.17 .07	.32 -.28	2.51** -2.40**
Patients with D & H	Future Orientation	.60	.37	.37	.60	.40**
Criterion = Adaptive Coping Strategies						
Cancer Patients	Optimism Psychological symptoms reported	.44 .59	.20 .34	.20 .14	.45 .38	3.22** 2.70**
Patients with D & H	Physical symptoms reported	.40	.18	.18	.43	2.73**
Criterion = Maladaptive Coping Strategies						
Cancer Patients	Physical symptoms reported	.7	.22	.22	.47	3.09**
Heart Patients	Optimism	.27	.07	.07	-.17	-2.09**
Criterion = Acceptance Coping Strategies						
Cancer Patients	Physical symptoms reported	.33	.11	.11	.33	2.04**
Criterion = Humour Coping Strategies						
Cancer Patients	Personal Control	.0	.16	.16	.40	2.51**
Diabetic Patients	Total Symptoms Reported	.34	.12	.12	-.34	-2.71**
Total Chronically Ill Group	Physical symptoms reported	.15	.025	.025	-.15	-2.13**
Healthy Group	Optimism	.26	.071	.071	.26	2.00**

Note: P<.01**, P<.05*.

variables together explained 48.8 per cent variance in the criterion variable. Relationship in family negatively explained 37.4 per cent variance, independently, followed by system maintenance in family which positively accounted for 11.3 per cent variance in the criterion variable, adaptive coping strategies (Table 9).

Table 9: Global Coping Strategies as Predicted by Social Variables in Patient and Healthy Groups

Group	Predictor	R	R^2	R^2 Change	Beta	t
Criterion= Combined Active Coping Strategies						
Cancer Patients	System maintenance in Family	.55	.30	.30	.53	3.82**
Heart Patients	Relationship in Family	.26	.07	.07	.26	2.16**
Patients with D & H	Personal growth in Family	.35	.12	.12	.35	2.18**
Criterion= Adaptive Coping Strategies						
Heart Patients	Relationship in Family	.37	.13	.13	.37	2.90**
Patients with D & H	Relationship in Family	.61	.37	.37	-.49	-3.64**
	System maintenance in Family	.69	.48	.13	.35	2.65**
Criterion= Maladaptive Coping Strategies						
Cancer Patients	Personal growth in Family	.39	.15	.15	.39	2.61**
Patients with D & H	Relationship in Family	.50	.25	.10	-.32	-2.84**
Criterion= Acceptance Coping Strategies						
Cancer Patients	System maintenance in Family	.17	.03	.03	-.17	-2.68**
Total Chronically Ill Group	System Maintenance in Family	.15	.025	.025	-.15	-2.12**
Criterion= Humour Coping Strategies						
Cancer Patients	System maintenance in Family	.13	.01	.01	.13	2.13**
Criterion= Adaptive Coping Strategies						
Healthy Group	Relationship in Family	.18	.03	.035	.30	3.80**
	Personal growth in Family	.30	.09	.060	-.27	-3.42**

Note: P<.01**, P<.05*

Adaptive Coping Strategies as Predicted by Psychosocial Variables: In chronically ill group of participants none of the psychosocial variables were significantly contributing in the prediction of using adaptive coping strategies. However, in healthy group of participants adaptive coping strategies were best predicted by a set of two social variables, namely, relationship in family and opportunities for personal growth in family [F(1,54) = 9.23, P<.000]. These two variables together explained 9.5 per cent of total variance in the criterion variable (Table 9).

Maladaptive Coping Strategies as Predicted by Psychosocial Variables: Table 10 shows that in chronically ill group of participants maladaptive coping strategies were significantly and negatively predicted by optimism [F(1,179) = 17.38, P<.000] which explained 8.9 per cent of total variance in the criterion variable. Table 10 reported that in healthy group of participants psychological symptoms reported [F (1, 54) = 13.24, P<.000] significantly predicted maladaptive coping strategies. Psychological symptoms reported explained 7.4 per cent variance in the criterion variable and it had a positive contribution.

Table 10: Psychological Variables as Predictors of Maladaptive Coping Strategies in Chronically Ill and Healthy Groups

Criterion = Maladaptive Coping					
Chronically Ill Group					
Predictors	R	R^2	R^2 Change	Beta	t
Optimism	.30	.089	.089	-.30	-4.16**
Healthy Group					
Psychological Symptoms Reported	.27	.07	.074	.27	3.77**

Note: P < .01**

In the different patient groups the prediction of psychosocial variables indicates that in cancer patient group of participants physical symptoms reported [F (1, 34) = 9.56, P<.004] positively predicted maladaptive coping strategies. Physical symptoms reported explained 22.5 per cent variance in the criterion, maladaptive coping strategies (Table 8). In cancer patient group of participants maladaptive coping strategies were also predicted by a set of two social variables, namely, personal growth in family [F (1, 34) = 5.58, P<.008]. Personal growth in family positively predicted 15.4 per cent variance. In diabetic patient group of participants maladaptive coping strategies were not significantly predicted by any psychosocial variables (Table 9).

In heart patients group participants maladaptive coping strategies were significantly and negatively predicted by optimism [F (1, 54) = 13.24, P<.001]. Optimism explained 7.6 per cent variance in the criterion variable (Table 8). In heart patients group of participants none of the social variable significantly explained maladaptive coping strategies.

In the group of patients suffering from both diabetes and heart problems maladaptive coping strategies were not significantly explained by any psychological variable. But it was significantly predicted by social variables, relationship in family [F(1,34) = 8.10, P<.008]. Relationship in family explained 19.7 per cent variance in the criterion variable (Table 9).

Acceptance Coping Strategy as Predicted by Psychosocial Variables: Table 9 shows that in chronically ill group of participants acceptance coping strategy was predicted by social variable, system maintenance in family [F(1,179) = 4.52, P<.03]. System maintenance in family negatively accounted for 2.5 per cent of variance in the criterion variable.

In cancer patients group of participants acceptance coping strategy was positively predicted by physical symptoms reported [F (1, 34) = 4.17, P<.04]. Physical symptoms reported explained 11.2 per cent variance in the criterion acceptance coping strategy (Table 8). In cancer patients group acceptance coping strategy was also significantly by negatively predicted by system maintenance in family explained 3 per cent variance in the use of acceptance coping strategy (Table 9). In diabetes patients, heart patients and patients suffering from both diabetes and heart problems none of the psychosocial variables significantly predicted acceptance coping strategy.

Humour Coping Strategy as Predicted by Psychosocial Variables: Table 8 reported that in chronically ill group of participants humour coping strategy was negatively predicted by physical symptoms reported [F(1,179) = 4.55, P<.03]. Physical symptoms reported explained 2.5 per cent of variance in the criterion variable.

In healthy group of participants humour coping strategy was positively and significantly predicted by optimism [F (1, 54) = 4.02, P<.05]. Optimism was responsible for 7.1 per cent of variance in explaining the criterion variable (Table 8). Use of humour coping strategy was not significantly predicted by any social variable in both chronically ill and healthy group of participants.

In cancer patient group of participants humour coping strategy was significantly and positively predicted personal control [F (1, 34) = 6.32, P<.01]. It explained 16.1 per cent variance in the criterion variable (Table 8). In cancer patients group humour coping strategy was also predicted by social variable, system maintenance in family [F (1, 34) = 2.13, P<.02]. System maintenance in family positively explained 13.8 per cent variance in the criterion variable (Table 9).

In diabetic patient group of participants humour coping strategy was significantly but negatively predicted by total symptoms reported [F (1, 54) = 5.09, P<.02]. Total symptoms reported explained 12.2 per cent variance in the criterion variable (Table 8). In this group none of the social variables predicted humour coping strategy.

In heart patients group and the group of patients suffering from both diabetes and heart problems humour coping strategy was not significantly predicted by any psychosocial variables.

Psychological Variables as Predictors of Different Components of Combined Active Coping, Adaptive Coping and Maladaptive Coping Strategies

Personal control predicted use of six coping strategies in chronically ill group of participants. Three of these can be classified into combined active coping strategies, one of these is adaptive and two of these are maladaptive coping strategies (Table 11). Personal control positively explained 7.4 per cent variance in positive reinterpretation coping strategy, 16.5 per cent variance in active coping strategy, 15.5 per cent in planning coping strategy. Physical symptoms reported by patients also negatively explained 3 per cent variance in planning coping strategy. Personal control negatively explained use of two maladaptive coping strategies, namely, mental disengagement and denial. It explained 14.1 per cent variance in the use of mental disengagement. Physical symptoms reported by patients also negatively explained 2.8 per cent variance in using mental disengagement. Personal control positively explained the use of denial coping strategy and accounted for 4.5 per cent of change in the use of denial coping strategy (Table 11).

Table 11: Components of Coping Strategies as Predicted by Psychological Variables in Chronically Ill Group

Criterion-Positive Reinterpretation					
Predictor	**R**	**R^2**	**R^2 Change**	**Beta**	**t**
Personal Control	.27	.074	.074	.27	3.77**
Criterion-Active Coping					
Personal Control	.406	.105	.165	.405	5.92**
Criterion-Planning					
Personal Control	.39	.155	.155	.377	5.53**
Physical Symptoms reported	.42	.187	.032	-.179	-2.62**
Criterion-Religion					
Personal Control	.27	.07	.07	-.27	-3.76**
Criterion-Mental Disengagement					
Personal Control	.37	.14	.14	-.39	-5.69**
Physical Symptoms reported	.41	.17	.028	-.16	-2.46**
Criterion-Denial					
Personal Control	.21	.04	.04	.21	2.88**
Criterion-Suppression of competing activities					
Future Orientation	.30	.09	.09	.30	4.27**
Criterion-Restraint Coping					
Future Orientation	.29	.085	.085	.29	3.17**
Optimism	.36	.132	.048	.22	3.13**
Criterion-Behavioural Disengagement					
Optimism	.11	.028	.028	-.16	-2.24**
Criterion-Venting off emotions					
Optimism	.33	.11	.11	-.32	-4.61**
Total symptoms reported	.39	.15	.04	.21	3.10**

Note: P<.01**, P<.05*

As opposed to this in healthy group of participants personal control predicted only one coping strategy behavioural disengagement, which is classified as maladaptive. Personal control positively explained 8.5 per cent variance in the use of behavioural disengagement (Table 12).

Table 12: Components of Coping Strategies as Predicted by Psychological Variables in Healthy Group

Criterion-Religion					
Predictor	**R**	R^2	R^2 **Change**	**Beta**	**t**
Future Orientation	.27	.07	.07	-.27	-2.04**
Criterion-Behavioural Disengagement					
Personal Control	.29	.08	.08	.29	2.21**
Criterion-Venting of emotions					
Optimism	.38	.15	.15	-.29	-2.34**
Total Symptoms reported	.48	.23	.08	.33	2.65**
Criterion-Instrumental Social support					
Total Symptoms reported	.27	.07	.07	.27	2.08**
Criterion-Positive Reinterpretation					
Psychological Symptoms reported	.28	.08	.08	.28	2.16**

Note: P<.01**, P<.05*

Future orientation predicted the use of two coping strategies in chronically ill group of participants and both of these are components of combined active coping strategies (Table 11). Future orientation positively explained 9.3 per cent variance in the use of suppression of competing activities and 8.5 per cent variance in restraint coping strategy. Optimism also positively explained 4.8 per cent variance in the use of restraint coping strategy (Table 11).

As opposed to this, in healthy group of participants future orientation predicted only one adaptive coping strategy, namely, religion (Table 12). Future orientation negatively accounted for 7.3 per cent variance in the use of religion coping strategy.

Optimism predicted lesser use of two maladaptive coping strategies in chronically ill group of participants. Optimism negatively explained 2.8 per cent variance in behavioural disengagement and 11.29 per cent variance in venting of emotions. Total symptoms reported by patients positively explained 4.6 per cent variance in venting of emotions (Table 11).

In healthy group of participants also one maladaptive coping strategy, namely, venting of emotions was negatively explained by optimism, which accounted for 15 per cent variance and total symptoms reported by participants positively predicted 8.1 per cent variance in the use of venting of emotions (Table 12). In healthy group of participants, on the other hand, total symptoms reported by participants predicted one adaptive coping strategy seeking instrumental social support. It positively explained 7.5 per cent variance. Psychological symptoms reported by participants positively predicted positive reinterpretation coping strategy in healthy group of participants, which accounted for 8.1 per cent variance (Table 12).

Social Variables as Predictors of Different Components of Combined Active Coping, Adaptive Coping and Maladaptive Coping Strategies

Relationship in family predicted four coping strategies in chronically ill group of participants (Table 13). Two of these were parts of combined active coping strategies. Relationship in family positively explained 10.8 per cent variance in active coping and 5 per cent variance in the use of positive reinterpretation coping strategy. Relationship in family also positively predicted 5.2 per cent variance in one adaptive coping strategy, namely, seeking instrumental social support. Opportunity for personal growth in family negatively explained 4.5 per cent variance in seeking instrumental social support. Relationship in family negatively predicted 9.7 per cent variance in the use of a maladaptive coping strategy, behavioural disengagement (Table 13).

System maintenance in family positively predicted two coping strategies in chronically ill group of participants (Table 13). These two coping strategies were components of combined active coping strategies. System maintenance in family explained 12 per cent variance in restraint coping and 2.2 per cent in the use of suppression of competing activities (Table 13).

In healthy group of participants none of the social variables were found as significant in explaining the change in the use of different coping strategies.

Coping Strategies and Quality of Life and Life Satisfaction

This section presents the relationship of five dimensions of quality of life, namely, physical, psychological, social, environmental and

Table 13: Components of Coping Strategies as Predicted by Social Variables in Chronically Ill Group

Criterion-Active coping					
Predictor	**R**	**R^2**	**R^2 Change**	**Beta**	**t**
Relationship in Family	.32	.10	.108	.32	4.64**
Criterion-Positive Reinterpretation					
Relationship in Family	.18	.05	.05	.18	2.49**
Criterion-Instrumental Social Support					
Relationship in Family	.23	.05	.05	.33	3.99**
Personal Growth in Family	.31	.09	.04	-.23	-2.83**
Criterion-Behavioural Disengagement					
Relationship in Family	.31	.09	.09	-.31	-4.19**
Criterion-Restraint coping					
Relationship in Family	.34	.12	.12	.34	4.92**
Criterion-Suppression of Competing Activities					
System maintenance in family	.15	.02	.02	.15	2.02**

Note: P<.01**, P<.05*

general health quality of life with different coping strategies and also the relationship of three temporal zones of satisfaction with life, namely, past, present and future satisfaction with life, as well as, total temporal satisfaction with life with different coping strategies. These analyses were computed in the light of the objective of the present investigation that effective coping strategies lead to better perception of quality of life and satisfaction with life. The significant coefficient of correlation between different coping strategies and quality of life and satisfaction with life are given in Table 14.

Coping Strategies as Predictors of Quality of Life and Life Satisfaction

Regression analyses were computed to investigate the role of different coping strategies in perception of quality of life and

Table 14: Coefficient of Correlation of Components of Global Coping Strategies and Quality of Life and Satisfaction with Life

Coping Strategies	Groups	Physical QOL	Psychological QOL	Social QOL	Environmental QOL	General Health QOL	Total QOL	Past SWL	Present SWL	Future SWL	Total SWL
Positive Reinterpretation	CIG	.21**	.26**	.27**	.13	.07	.13	-.07	.35**	.23**	.24**
	HG	.12	-.13	.08	.03	.28**	.26	-.09	.13	.08	.03
Planning	CIG	.19**	.28**	.39**	-.22**	.03	-.12	.05	.24**	.36**	.34**
	HG	-.14	.20	.05	.07	.02	-.27**	.16	.04	.01	.14
Active Coping	CIG	.22**	.24**	.41**	-.14	-.12	-.17*	.04	.38**	.31**	.35**
	HG	-.05	-.05	.16	.05	-.09	-.06	-.10	.03	.04	-.03
Restraint Coping	CIG	.29**	.29**	.20**	-.08	-.07	-.10	-.08	.33**	.31**	.23**
	HG	.32*	.12	.22	-.12	-.14	-.18	.09	.06	.21	.21
Suppression of Competing Activities	CIG	.16**	.31**	.24**	.06	.09	.04	-.06	.25**	.28**	.23**
	HG	.02	-.03	.13	-.03	-.07	-.01	-.09	.21	.15	.10
Combined Active Coping	CIG	.34**	.43**	.46**	-.15*	-.12	-.18*	-.04	.48**	.46**	.44**
	HG	.12	.01	.24	.009	.01	.02	-.01	.18	.21	.18
Religion	CIG	-.18*	-.15*	-.27**	.10	.13	.15*	.02	-.10	-.13	-.10
	HG	.05	-.27*	.003	.03	.14	.13	.01	.15	-.06	.09
Instrumental Social Support	CIG	.15*	.16*	.05	-.06	.09	.03	-.04	.08	.07	.05
	HG	-.02	.04	.01	.17	.22	.27	-.26	-.08	-.03	-.17

(*Contd.*)

(*Contd.*)

Emotional Social Support	CIG	-.08	.03	-.04	.08	.04	.08	.01	.02	-.03	.01
	HG	-.18	-.18	-.26	.21	.02	.12	.08	-.08	-.19	-.09
Adaptive Coping	CIG	-.03	.04	-.09	.05	.12	.11	-.04	.01	-.02	-.01
	HG	-.06	-.18	-.10	.18	.17	.23	-.08	.07	-.06	-.07
Venting of emotions	CIG	-.33**	-.11	-.14	.21**	.15**	.24**	.09	-.11	-.17**	.09
	HG	-.36**	-.34**	-.39**	.16	.36**	.39**	.14	.09	-.52**	-.19
Mental disengage-ment	CIG	-.14	.25**	-.38**	-.13	-.02	.21	.01	.01	-.34**	-.18*
	HG	.02	-.23	.22	.04	.21	.26**	-.09	.17	-.03	-.02
Behavioural disengagement	CIG	-.17*	.15	-.02	.13	-.09	.03	.05	.03	.12	.11
	HG	-.06	.02	-.01	.11	.28**	.29**	.01	.15	.03	.08
Denial	CIG	.05	.05	.21**	.01	-.10	-.06	.01	.08	.01	.05
	HG	.14	.18	.16	-.11	.14	-.02	-.23	-.20	.11	-.16
Maladaptive Coping	CIG	-.30**	-.11	-.18**	.12	-.03	.05	.08	.01	-.16*	-.04
	HG	-.16	-.19	-.13	.20	.45**	.44**	-.05	.10	-.25*	-.15
Acceptance Coping	CIG	.04	.08	.04	.07	-.07	.01	.13	-.03	.01	.06
	HG	.16	-.14	.17	-.17	-.01	-.19	.08	-.01	.26*	.22*
Humour Coping	CIG	-.02	.04	.09	-.15*	-.17	-.15*	-.23**	.05	.02	-.08
	HG	.66**	.06	.12	-.25	-.01	-.13	-.18	-.07	.17	-.04

satisfaction with life. Different coping strategies were chosen as predictors, to predict the quality of life and satisfaction with life in chronically ill and healthy group of participants. In the first stance all components of active, adaptive and maladaptive coping strategies were combined to give one score each of active, adaptive and maladaptive coping strategies, respectively. These scores, and acceptance and *humour* coping were entered as predictors.

Total Quality of Life as Predicted by Coping Strategies: In chronically ill group of participants total quality of life was significantly predicted by two coping strategies, namely, combined active coping and maladaptive coping strategies [F(1,179) = 22.49, P<.000]. These two variables together explained 20.3 per cent of total variance in the criterion variable. Combined active coping strategies positively predicted total quality of life, whereas, maladaptive coping strategies negatively predicted total quality of life. Combined active coping strategies constituted the best predictor which explained 15.8 per cent of total variance in this criterion variable independently, followed by, maladaptive coping strategies which accounted for 4.5 per cent variance in the criterion variable (Table 15).

Table 15: Psychological Variables as Predictors of Total Quality of Life in Chronically Ill Group

Criterion = Total Quality of Life					
Predictors	**R**	**R^2**	**R^2 Change**	**Beta**	**t**
Combined Active Coping	.31	.16	.158	-.37	5.49**
Maladaptive Coping	.45	.20	.045	-.21	-3.15**

Note: P<.01**

Table 15 shows that quality of life was significantly predicted by different components of combined active coping, adaptive and maladaptive coping strategies in both chronically ill and healthy group of participants. In chronically ill group of participants two components of combined active coping strategies, namely, active coping and suppression of competing activities [F(1,179) = 19.18, P<.00] significantly and positively predicted total quality of life. These two variables together explained 17.9 per cent of total variance in the criterion variable. Active coping was the best predictor which explained 12.2 per cent of total variance in the criterion variable, independently, followed by suppression of competing activities which accounted for 7.5 per cent of variance in the criterion.

Table 16: Components of Coping Strategies as Predictors of Total Quality of Life in Chronically Ill and Healthy Groups

Criterion = Total Quality of Life					
Chronically Ill Group					
Predictors	**R**	**R^2**	**R^2 Change**	**Beta**	**t**
Active Coping	.35	.12	.122	.25	3.61**
Suppression of competing activities	.42	.18	.057	.25	3.49**
Religion	.23	.05	.051	-.22	-3.08**
Behavioural Disengagement	.27	.070	.070	-.24	-3.33**
Venting of Emotions	.35	.12	.051	-.22	-3.20**
Healthy Group					
Behavioural Disengagement	.29	.08	.085	-.29	-2.21**

Note: P<.01**

Table 16 shows that in chronically ill group of participants adaptive coping strategy, religion significantly and negatively predicted total quality of life [F(1,179) = 9.50, P,<.00]. Religion explained 5.1 per cent variance in the criterion variable. Similarly, two components of maladaptive coping strategies, namely, behavioural disengagement and venting of emotions [F(1,179) = 12.21, P<.002] predicted total quality of life. These two variables together explained 12.1 per cent total variance in the criterion variables. Behavioural disengagement explained 7 per cent variance independently, followed by venting of emotions which accounted for 5.1 per cent variance in the criterion variables. In healthy group of participants also maladaptive coping strategy, behavioural disengagement significantly and negatively predicted total quality of life [F (1, 54) = 4.89, P<.002] (Table 16).

Coping Strategies as Predictors of Total Quality of Life in Different Patient Groups: Total quality of life as predicted by coping [*Note*: P<.01**] strategies in four patient groups, separately, was presented in Table 17. This table shows that in cancer patient group of participants combined active coping strategies significantly and positively predicted total quality of life [F(1,34) = 9.38, P<.004].

Combined active coping strategies explained 22 per cent variance in the criterion variable. In diabetic patient group of participants total quality of life was predicted by maladaptive coping strategies which explained 13.7 per cent variance in the criterion variable. It had negative contribution in the criterion variable. In heart patient group of participants combined active coping strategies [F (1, 54) = 13.71, P<.001] significantly and positively predicted total quality of life. Combined active coping strategies explained 20.6 per cent variance in the criterion variable (Table 17). In the group of patients afflicted with both diabetes and heart problems two coping strategies, namely, adaptive coping and maladaptive coping strategies [F (1, 34) = 19.18, P<.000] significantly predicted total quality of life. These two coping strategies together explained 54.4 per cent variance in the criterion variable. Adaptive coping strategies explained 44.1 per cent variance in the criterion variable independently, followed by, maladaptive coping strategies which accounted for 10.4 per cent variance in the criterion variable. Both of these coping strategies had negative contribution in the prediction of total quality of life.

Table 17: Coping Strategies as Predictors of Quality of Life in Different Patient Groups

Groups	*Predictors*	*R*	R^2	R^2 *Change*	*Beta*	*t*
Cancer Patients	Combined Active Coping	.47	.22	.221	.47	3.06**
Heart Patients	Combined Active Coping	.45	.20	.206	.45	3.70**
Diabetic Patients	Maladaptive Coping	.37	.13	.137	-.37	-2.90**
Patients with D&H	Adaptive Coping	.66	.44	.441	-.33	-4.78**
	Maladaptive Coping	.73	.54	.104	-.58	-2.70**

Note: P<.01**, P<.05*

Coping Strategies as Predictors of Domains of Quality of Life: Table 18 shows the variance in different domains of quality of life, namely, physical quality of life, psychological quality of life, social quality of life, environmental quality of life and general health quality of life as predicted by combined active coping, adaptive coping, maladaptive coping strategies, as well as, different components of it.

Table 18: Coping Strategies as Predictors of Quality of Life in Different Domains

Chronically Ill Group					
Criterion = Physical Quality of Life					
Predictors	**R**	**R^2**	**R^2 Change**	**Beta**	**t**
Combined Active Coping	.28	.08	.082	.20	4.29**
Acceptance Coping	.34	.11	.034	-.18	-2.62**
Venting of Emotions	.22	.04	.048	-.20	-2.74**
Behavioural Disengagement	.27	.07	.023	-.15	-2.08**
Suppression of Competing Activities	.27	.05	.052	.22	3.06**
Planning	.27	.07	.024	.15	2.15**
Criterion = Psychological Quality of Life					
Suppression of Competing Activities	.23	.10	.105	.24	3.29**
Active Coping	.39	.15	.050	.23	3.22**
Religion	.20	.04	.044	-.20	-2.85**
Behavioural Disengagement	.26	.06	.068	-.23	-3.31**
Venting of Emotions	.31	.10	.032	-.18	-2.51**
Criterion = Social Quality of Life					
Active Coping	.27	.07	.073	.27	3.73**
Religion	.21	.04	.046	-.22	-2.98**
Seeking Instrumental Social Support	.29	.08	.029	-.17	-2.27**
Venting of Emotions	.22	.05	.052	-.20	-2.69**
Behavioural Disengagement	.28	.08	.029	-.17	-2.24**
Criterion = Environmental Quality of Life					
Active Coping	.20	.04	.040	.26	3.41**
Positive Reinterpretation	.26	.07	.030	-.18	-2.40**
Planning	.33	.10	.109	.29	4.28**
Restraint Coping	.42	.17	.069	.26	3.35**
Mental Disengagement	.37	.13	.139	-.37	-5.35**
Combined Active Coping	.39	.15	.158	.37	5.51**
Maladaptive Coping	.42	.18	.026	-.16	2.39**

(Contd.)

Healthy Group					
Criterion = Social Quality of Life					
Behavioural Disengagement	.28	.08	.081	-.28	-2.15**
Emotional Social Support	.33	.11	.115	.33	2.62**
Criterion = Environmental Quality of Life					
Humour	.35	.12	.123	-3.15	-2.72**

Table 18 shows that in chronically ill group of participants combined active coping strategies predicted 8.2 per cent variance, in physical quality of life. Acceptance coping strategy also accounted for 3.4 per cent variance in physical quality of life. Two maladaptive coping strategies, namely, venting of emotions and behavioural disengagement negatively predicted three domains of quality of life, like, physical, psychological and social quality of life. Venting of emotions explained 4.8 per cent variance in physical quality of life, 3.2 per cent variance in psychological quality of life and 5.2 per cent variance in social quality of life. Behavioural disengagement coping strategy explained 2.3 per cent variance in physical quality, 6.8 per cent variance in psychological quality of life and 2.9 per cent variance in social quality of life. As opposed to this in healthy group of participants behavioural disengagement coping strategy negatively explained 8.1 per cent variance in social quality of life, where seeking emotional social support also accounted for 11.5 per cent positive variance in social quality of life.

Table 18 also shows that component of combined active coping strategy, suppression of competing activities explained 5.2 per cent variance in physical quality of life, where planning also explained 2.4 per cent variance and 10.5 per cent variance in psychological quality of life. Planning also explained 10.9 per cent variance in general health quality of life, where, restraint coping accounted 6.9 per cent variance in general health quality of life. Active coping strategy explained 5 per cent variance in social quality of life and 4 per cent variance in environmental quality of life, where, positive reinterpretation also explained 3 per cent variance.

Table 18 presents that in chronically ill group of participants' adaptive coping strategy, religion predicted two domains of quality of life, namely, psychological quality of life and social quality of life. Religion explained 4.4 per cent variance in psychological quality of life and 4.6 per cent variance in social quality of life. Seeking instrumental social support also accounted for 4 per cent variance in social quality of life.

Table 18 also reveals that in chronically ill group of participants maladaptive coping strategy mental disengagement negatively explained 13.9 per cent variance in prediction of general health quality of life.

Table 18 presents that environmental quality of life was significantly predicted by *humour* as a coping strategy. *Humour* coping strategy explained 12.3 per cent variance in environmental quality of life.

Coping Strategies as Predictors of Total Temporal Satisfaction with Life: Table 19 reported that in chronically ill group of participants total temporal satisfaction with life was best predicted by a set of two coping strategies, viz. combined active coping and humour coping strategies [F(1,179) = 26.30, P<.000]. These two predictors together explained 22.9 per cent of total variance in the criterion variable. Combined active coping strategies explained 19.6 per cent of total variance in the criterion variable, independently, followed by humour coping strategy which accounted for 3.3 per cent variance in the criterion variable. Combined active coping strategies positively contributed in explaining the variance in criterion variable, whereas, humour coping strategy had a negative contribution in explaining the criterion variable. In healthy group of participants none of these coping strategies predicted significant variance in criterion variable.

Table 19: Coping Strategies as Predictors of Total Temporal Satisfaction with Life in Chronically Ill Group

Criterion = Total Temporal Satisfaction with Life					
Predictors	**R**	**R^2**	**R^2 Change**	**Beta**	**t**
Combined Active Coping	.44	.19	.196	.49	7.07**
Humour Coping	.46	.22	.033	-.16	-2.36**

Note: P<.01**,

Table 20: Components of Combined Active Coping Strategies as Predictors of Total Temporal Satisfaction with Life in Chronically Ill Group

Criterion = Total Temporal Satisfaction with Life					
Predictors	**R**	**R^2**	**R^2 Change**	**Beta**	**t**
Active Coping	.35	.15	.125	.23	3.23**
Planning	.42	.17	.051	.22	3.17**
Restraint Coping	.45	.20	.033	.18	2.69**

Note: P<.01**, P<.05*

Table 20 presents that in chronically ill group of participants total temporal satisfaction with life was positively predicted by a set of three components of combined active coping strategies, namely, active coping, planning and restraint coping [F(1,179) = 15.45, P<000]. These three variables together explained 20.9 per cent variance in the criterion variable. Active coping explained 12.5 per cent of total variance in the criterion variable, independently, followed by planning coping strategy which accounted for 5.1 per cent variance in the criterion variable, then comes restraint coping strategy which was found responsible for 3.3 per cent of variance in the criterion variable.

Coping strategies as Predictors of Total Temporal Satisfaction with Life in Different Patients Groups: Predictive power of coping strategies in different patient groups were also analyzed separately which is shown in Table 21. This table presents that in cancer patient group of participants combined active strategies and humour coping strategy [F(1,34) = 11.41, P<.000] significantly predicted total temporal satisfaction with life. These two variables together explained 41.7 per cent variance in the criterion variable. Active coping strategy explained 25.9 per cent variance, independently, followed by humour coping strategy, which accounted for 15.8 per cent variance in the criterion variable. Examination of beta value suggest that combined active coping strategies positively contributing in the criterion variable, whereas, humour coping strategy had negative contribution in explaining total temporal satisfaction with life.

Table 21: Coping Strategies as Predictors of Temporal Satisfaction with Life in Different Patient Groups

Groups	Predictors	R	R^2	R^2 change	Beta	t
Cancer Patients	Combined Active Coping	.50	.25	.259	.58	4.24**
	Humour Coping	.64	.41	.158	-.40	-2.94**
Diabetic Patients	Combined Active Coping	.34	.11	.116	.34	2.63**
Heart Patients	Combined Active Coping	.56	.31	.317	.56	4.95**
Patients with D&H	Adaptive Coping	.33	.11	.11	-.33	-2.04**

Note: P<.01

In diabetic patient group of participants only combined coping strategy positively predicted total temporal satisfaction, with life [F(1,54) = 6.95, P<.01] (Table 21). Combined active coping explained 11.6 per cent variance in the criterion variable. In heart patient group of participants combined active coping strategy positively predicted total temporal satisfaction with life [F(1,54) = 24.59, P<.000]. Combined active coping strategies accounted for 31.7 per cent of total variance. In the group of patients suffering from both diabetes and heart problems adaptive coping strategies was negatively predicted total temporal satisfaction with life [F (1, 54) = 4.16, P<.04] (Table 21).

Coping Strategies as Predictors of Different Time Zones (Past, Present, Future) of Temporal Satisfaction with Life: Another regression analysis was computed to examine the role of different components of active, adaptive and maladaptive coping strategies, in predicting three time zones (past, present and future) of satisfaction with life.

Table 22 shows that in chronically ill group of participants combined active coping strategies positively explained 23.2 per cent variance in satisfaction with present life and 21.1 per cent variance in satisfaction with future life and adaptive coping strategies negatively explained 2.1 per cent variance in satisfaction with present life and 3.2 per cent variance in satisfaction with future life (Table 22). In chronically ill group of participants three components of combined active coping strategies also significantly and positively predicted satisfaction with present life. Active coping explained 13.9 per cent variance, restraint coping explained 6.5 per cent variance and positive reinterpretation accounted for 2.9 per cent variance in satisfaction with present life. In this group satisfaction with past life was significantly and negatively predicted by humour coping strategy, which explained 5.3 per cent variance in the criterion variable (Table 22). As opposed to this in healthy group of participants' maladaptive coping strategy, i.e., venting of emotions negatively predicted satisfaction with future life. It explained 27.8 per cent variance in satisfaction with future life. None of the active and adaptive coping strategies predicted past, present and future satisfaction life in healthy group of participants.

Table 22: Coping Strategies as Predictors of Temporal Satisfaction with Life in Different Time Zones

Chronically Ill Group					
Criterion = Past Satisfaction with Life					
Predictors	**R**	**R^2**	**R^2 Change**	**Beta**	**t**
Humour Coping	.23	.053	.053	-.230	-3.15**
Criterion = Present Satisfaction with Life					
Combined Active Coping	.48	.23	.232	.28	7.13**
Adaptive Coping	.50	.25	.021	-.15	-2.22**
Active Coping	.37	.13	.139	.26	3.77**
Restraint Coping	.45	.20	.065	.20	2.82**
Positive Reinterpretation	.48	.23	.029	.19	2.58**
Criterion = Future Satisfaction with Life					
Combined Active Coping	.45	.21	.211	.51	7.52**
Adaptive Coping	.49	.24	.032	-.18	-2.72**
Healthy Group					
Criterion = Future Satisfaction with Life					
Venting of Emotions	.52	.27	.278	-.52	-4.51**

Note: P<.01**, P<.05*

SECTION-C

In this section of results the relationship between psychosocial characteristics of the participants and perception of quality of life has been presented.

Quality of Life of Participants: Table 23 presents the means and standard deviations of quality of life in various domains of life, i.e. physical, psychological, social, environmental and general health quality of life as perceived by chronically ill, healthy and total group of participants. Table 27 reveals that healthy group of participants perceive their quality of life in a better way than chronically ill group of participants in all domains of life.

Table 23: Means and Standard Deviations of Quality of Life

Quality of Life	*Cancer Patients*	*Diabetic Patients*	*Heart Patients*	*Patients with both D&H*	*Healthy Group*
Physical QOL	86.68 (10.10)	89.70 (7.38)	91.90 (8.25)	86.05 (7.38)	102.10 (7.36)
Psychological QOL	76.20 (13.29)	81.45 (6.90)	83.67 (13.29)	78.40 (9.61)	91.40 (9.49)
Social QOL	41.08 (6.46)	44.54 (4.80)	42.01 (5.31)	40.02 (6.28)	47.25 (5.86)
Environmental QOL	88.45 (9.41)	92.41 (13.68)	96.45 (13.59)	90.34 (9.70)	99.58 (8.02)
General Health QOL	13.00 (3.34)	13.98 (2.71)	14.58 (2.95)	13.74 (2.22)	16.89 (3.08)
Total QOL	**293.17 (38.96)**	**311.14 (20.65)**	**314.94 (34.93)**	**296.62 (26.65)**	**349.05 (26.78)**

Note: Standard Deviations in parentheses.

Correlation between Psychosocial Variables and Quality of Life

The correlations amongst all the psychosocial variables under investigation and domains of QOL have been presented in Tables 24 and 25.

Psychosocial Variables as Predictors of Quality of Life

To understand the contribution of psychosocial variables in predicting the perception of quality of life in different domains SMRA were made. In regression analysis two sets of predictors were entered separately to domains of quality of life, as well as, total quality of life. The two sets of predictors were (i) psychological variables optimism, future orientation, personal control and symptoms reported by participants, (ii) social variables—relationship in family, opportunities for personal growth in family and system maintenance in family.

Table 24: Coefficient of Correlation of Psychological Variables and QOL

Quality of Life	*Groups*	*Optimism*	*Future Orientation*	*Perceived Control*	*Physical Symptoms Reported*	*Psychological Symptoms Reported*	*Total Symptoms Reported*
Physical QOL	CIG	19**	.06	.18**	-.08	.00	-.05
	HG	.03	-.10	-.00	.12	-.29**	-.19
Psychological QOL	CIG	.26**	.17**	.32**	-.13	-.05	-.12
	HG	.07	-.13	-.09	.20	-.04	.05
Social QOL	CIG	.05	.04	.03	-.33**	-.03	-.24**
	HG	.01	-.11	-.05	.04	-.24	-.19
Environmental QOL	CIG	.08	-.04	.07	-.05	.02	-.01
	HG	-.01	-.12	-.01	.16	-.00	.06
General Health QOL	CIG	.27**	.49**	.56**	-.13	.01	-.07
	HG	.34**	.55**	.82**	-.17	-.36**	-.39**
Total QOL	CIG	.27**	.19**	.33**	-.19*	-.04	-.15*
	HG	.01	.08	.01	.16	.20	-.10

Note: P<.01**, P<.05*

Table 25: Coefficient of Correlation of Social Variables and QOL

Quality of Life	*Groups*	*Relationship in Family*	*Personal Growth in Family*	*System Maintenance in Family*
Physical QOL	CIG	.20**	.05	.20**
	HG	.38**	-.12	.07
Psychological QOL	CIG	.31**	.14	.30**
	HG	.18	.07	.19
Social QOL	CIG	.35**	.26**	.13
	HG	.40**	-.11	.10
Environmental QOL	CIG	.18**	.17*	.17*
	HG	.32**	-.05	-.08
General Health QOL	CIG	.27**	.19**	.23**
	HG	.20**	-.08	.19
Total QOL	CIG	.36**	.19*	.31**
	HG	.33**	.00	.19

Note: P<.01**, P<.05*

Physical Quality of Life as Predicted by Psychosocial Variables: Table 26 presents the results of the SMRA in chronically ill group of participants which identified the best predictor of physical quality of life, i.e. optimism [F(1,179) = 7.12, P<.008]. Optimism positively explained 3.9 per cent of variance in the criterion variable independently. Table 26 presents that in chronically ill group of participants physical quality of life was also predicted by a social factor, system maintenance in family [F(1, 179) = 9.99, P<.002]. System maintenance in family positively explained 5.3 per cent of total variance in this criterion variable. In healthy group of participants physical quality of life was predicted by psychological symptoms reported [F (1, 54) = 5.185, P<.02]. Psychological symptoms reported negatively explained 8.9 per cent of variance in the criterion variable. In healthy group physical quality of life was also predicted by social variable relationship in family [F (1, 54) = 8.380, P<.005]. Relationship in family was positively explained 13.7 per cent variance in the criterion variable (Table 27).

Psychological Quality of Life as Predicted by Psychosocial Variables: Table 26 presents that in chronically ill group of participants psychological quality of life was significantly and positively predicted by two variables, namely, personal control and optimism [F(1,179) = 12.68, P<.000]. These two variables together explained 12.6 per cent of total variance in the criterion variable. Personal control explained 10.1 per cent of total variance in the criterion variable independently, followed by optimism, which accounted for 2.5 per cent of variance in the criterion variable. Table 27 shows that in chronically ill group of participants psychological quality of life was also significantly predicted by social factors, relationship in family and system maintenance in family [F(1,179) = 13.41, P<.000]. These two variables together positively explained 13.1 per cent of variance in the criterion variable. Relationship in family was the best predictor, which explained 9.4 per cent of variance in the criterion variable, independently, followed by system maintenance in family, which accounted for 3.7 per cent of variance. In healthy group of participants psychological quality of life was not significantly predicted by any of the psychosocial variables.

Social Quality of Life as Indicated by Psychosocial Variables: Table 26 shows that in chronically ill group of participants social quality of life was best predicted by physical symptoms reported [F(1, 179) = 22.74, P<.000]. Physical symptoms reported negatively explained 10.9 per cent of total variance in the criterion variable.

Table 26: Psychological Variables as Predictors of QOL in Different Domains

Chronically ill Group					
Criterion = Psychological QOL					
Predictors	**R**	**R^2**	**R^2 Change**	**Beta**	**t**
Personal Control	.31	.10	.101	.25	3.45**
Optimism	.35	.12	.025	.16	2.23**
Criterion = Physical QOL					
Optimism	.19	.03	.039	.19	2.67**
Criterion = Social QOL					
Physical Symptoms Reported	.33	.01	.019	-.33	-4.66**
Criterion = General Health QOL					
Personal Control	.56	.31	.312	.42	5.53**
Optimism	.59	.35	.351	.22	2.98**
Criterion = Total QOL					
Personal Control	.37	.13	.027	.17	2.35**
Optimism	.33	.11	.111	.27	3.61**
Healthy Group					
Criterion = Physical QOL					
Psychological Symptoms Reported	.29	.08	.089	-.29	-2.27**
Criterion = General Health QOL					
Personal Control	.82	.68	.684	.82	10.70**

Note: P<.01**, P<.05*

Table 27 presents that in chronically ill group of participants social variable of relationship in family was the best predictor [F (1,179) = 24.59, P<.000]. Relationship in family positively explained 12.1 per cent of total variance in the criterion variable.

Table 27 presents that in the healthy group of participants also relationship in family positively predicted social quality of life [F(1,54) = 10.39, P<.000], which accounted for 16.3 per cent of variance in the criterion variable. In the healthy group of participants none of the psychological variables significantly contributed in explaining social quality of life.

Table 27: Social Variables as Predictors of QOL in Different Domains

Predictors	R	R^2	R^2 Change	Beta	t
Chronically ill Group					
Criterion = Physical QOL					
System Maintenance in Family	.23	.05	.053	.23	3.16**
Criterion = Psychological QOL					
Relationship in Family	.30	.09	.094	.22	2.94**
System Maintenance in Family	.36	.13	.037	.21	2.76**
Criterion = Social QOL					
Relationship in Family	.37	.12	.121	.34	4.96**
Criterion = Environmental QOL					
Relationship in Family	.18	.03	.033	.18	2.46**
Criterion = General Health QOL					
Relationship in Family	.20	.04	.041	.28	4.62**
Personal Growth in Family	.27	.07	.033	-.20	-2.53**
Criterion = Total QOL					
Relationship in Family	.35	.12	.126	.27	3.65**
System Maintenance in Family	.40	.16	.036	.20	2.76**
Healthy Group					
Criterion = Physical QOL					
Relationship in Family	.37	.13	.137	.37	2.89**
Criterion = Social QOL					
Relationship in Family	.40	.16	.163	.40	3.21**
Criterion = Environmental QOL					
Relationship in Family	.32	.10	.105	.32	2.49**
Criterion = Total QOL					
Relationship in Family	.32	.10	.106	.32	2.50**

Note: P<.01**, P<.05*

Environmental Quality of Life as Predicted by Psychosocial Variables: Table 27 shows that in chronically ill group of participants environmental quality of life was significantly and positively predicted by social factor, relationship in family, [F(1,179) = 6.06, P<.01], which accounted for 3.3 per cent of total variance in the criterion variable.

Table 27 reported that in healthy group of participants also environmental quality of life was significantly predicted by social factor, relationship in family [F(1,54) = 6.231, P<.01]. Relationship in family positively explained 10.5 per cent of total variance in the criterion variable. None of the psychological variables significantly contributed in predicting environmental quality of life in both chronically ill and healthy group of participants.

General Health Quality of Life as Predicted by Psychosocial Variables: Table 26 shows that in chronically ill group of participants two predictors personal control and future orientation, [F(1,179) = 47.761, P<.000] positively predicted general health quality of life. These two variables together explained 35.1 per cent of total variance in the criterion variable. Personal control explained 31.3 per cent of total variance in the criterion variable independently, followed by future orientation, which accounted for 3.9 per cent of variance in the criterion variable. Table 26 shows that in healthy group of participants general health quality of life was significantly and positively predicted by personal control [F(1,54) = 114.59, P<.000]. Personal control explained 68.4 per cent of total variance in the criterion variable. Table 27 shows that in chronically ill group of participants general health quality of life was significantly predicted by social factors, viz. relationship in family and opportunities for personal growth in family [F(1,179) = 7.17, P<.001]. These two variables together explained 7.4 per cent of total variance in the criterion variable. Relationship in family positively explained 4.1 per cent of total variance in the criterion variable independently, followed by opportunities for personal growth, which negatively accounted for 3.3 per cent of variance in the criterion variable.

Total Quality of Life as Predicted by Psychosocial Variables: Table 26 shows that in chronically ill group of participants total quality of life was significantly predicted by a set of two variables, namely, personal control and optimism [F(1,179) = 14.11, P<.000]. These two variables positively explained 13.8 per cent of variance in the criterion variable. Personal control was the best predictor, which explained 11.1

per cent of variance in the criterion variable, independently, followed by optimism, which accounted for 2.7 per cent variance in the criterion variable.

Table 27 shows that in chronically ill group of participants total quality of life was positively predicted by two social variables, viz. relationship in family and system maintenance in family [$F(1,179) = 17.12$, $P<.000$]. These two variables together explained 16.2 per cent variance in the criterion variable. Relationship in family was the best predictor which explained 12.6 per cent variance in the criterion independently, followed by system maintenance in family, which accounted for 3.6 per cent in the criterion variable. Table 31 shows that in healthy group of participants also relationship in family positively predicted total quality of life [$F\ (1, 54) = 6.629$, $P<.01$]. Relationship in family explained 10.6 per cent of total variance in the criterion variable.

Psychosocial Variables as Predictors of Total Quality of Life in Different Patient Groups: Table 28 shows that in diabetic patient group of participants personal control had significantly and positively predicted total quality of life [$F(1,54) = 12.69$, $P<.000$]. Personal control explained 16 per cent variance in the criterion variable. In heart patient group of participants personal control significantly and positively predicted total quality of life [$F\ (1, 54) = 6.68$, $P<.000$]. Personal control explained 15 per cent variance in the criterion variable. In the group of patients afflicted with both diabetes and heart diseases physical symptoms reported [$F\ (1, 34) = 36.70$, $P<.000$] significantly and negatively predicted total quality of life. It explained 24.3 per cent variance in the criterion variable.

Table 28 shows that in diabetic patient group of participants personal control had significantly and positively predicted total quality of life [$F(1,54) = 12.69$, $P<.000$]. Personal control explained 16 per cent variance in the criterion variable. In heart patient group of participants personal control significantly and positively predicted total quality of life [$F\ (1, 54) = 6.68$, $P<.000$]. Personal control explained 15 per cent variance in the criterion variable. In the group of patients afflicted with both diabetes and heart diseases physical symptoms reported [$F\ (1, 34) = 36.70$, $P<.000$] significantly and negatively predicted total quality of life. It explained 24.3 per cent variance in the criterion variable.

Table 28: Psychosocial Variables as Predictors of QOL in Different Patient Groups

Groups	Predictors	R	R^2	R^2 Change	Beta	t
Psychological Variables						
Diabetic Patients	Personal Control	.40	.16	.160	.40	3.17**
Heart Patients	Personal Control	.38	.15	.150	.38	3.05**
Patients with both Diabetes and Heart	Physical Symptoms Reported	.49	.24	.243	-.49	3.25**
Social Variables						
Cancer Patients	System Maintenance in Family	.52	.27	.278	.52	3.56**
Heart Patients	System Maintenance in Family	.33	.11	.11	.32	2.58**
Patients with both Diabetes and Heart	Relationship in Family	.72	.52	.52	.76	6.05**

SECTION-D

This section presents the relationship between psychosocial variables and satisfaction with life.

Satisfaction with Life of Participants: Table 29 presents the means and standard deviations of satisfaction with life in different time zones, i.e. past, present and future. There were mean differences in satisfaction with past, present and future life, as well as, total temporal satisfaction with life in chronically ill and healthy group of participants.

Table 29: Means and Standard Deviations of Satisfaction with Life

Satisfaction with Life	*Cancer Patients*	*Diabetic Patients*	*Heart Patients*	*Patients with both D&H*	*Healthy Group*
Past SWL	19.80 (8.83)	19.78 (5.90)	22.00 (5.53)	20.85 (6.17)	19.36 (5.63)
Present SWL	18.38 (7.00)	20.38 (4.82)	22.07 (4.52)	18.45 (3.95)	24.83 (3.02)
Future SWL	21.14 (8.19)	21.78 (7.40)	20.45 (6.98)	21.85 (6.13)	28.81 (5.32)
Total SWL	56.62 (15.88)	61.92 (12.05)	64.62 (10.69)	61.77 (10.94)	73.01 (8.66)

Note: Standard Deviations in parentheses.

Psychosocial Variables and Life Satisfaction

The correlations amongst all the psychosocial variables under investigation and domains of SWL have been presented in Tables 30 and 31.

Table 30: Coefficient of Correlation of Psychological Variables and SWL

Satisfaction with Life	*Groups*	*Optimism*	*Future Orientation*	*Perceived Control*	*Physical Symptoms Reported*	*Psychological Symptoms Reported*	*Total Symptoms Reported*
Past SWL	CIG	-.05	-.05	-.00	.04	.00	.07
	HG	-.06	-.02	-.21	-.06	-.05	.05
Present SWL	CIG	.28**	.35**	.34**	-.22**	-.07	-.18**
	HG	.06	-.09	.17	-.04	.00	-.01
Future SWL	CIG	.23**	.56**	.65**	-.09	-.16*	-.17*
	HG	.51**	.58**	.69**	-.12	-.33**	-.35**
Total SWL	CIG	.22**	.44**	.51**	-.12**	-.09	-.14
	HG	.37**	.38**	.41**	-.14**	-.36**	-.37**

Note: P<.01**

Table 31: Coefficient of Correlation of Social Variables and SWL

Satisfaction with Life	*Groups*	*Relationship in Family*	*Personal Growth in Family*	*System Maintenance in Family*
Past SWL	CIG	-.06	.08	-.01
	HG	-.01	-.09	.63**
Present SWL	CIG	.30**	.11	.06
	HG	.21	.06	-.05
Future SWL	CIG	.06	.05	.12
	HG	.02	-.03	-.03
Total SWL	CIG	.19	.06	.13
	HG	.04	-.03	-.09

Note: P<.01**

Psychosocial Variables as Predictors of Life Satisfaction

To understand the role of psychosocial variables in predicting greater satisfaction within different time zones, i.e. past, present and, future life SMRA were computed. In these analyses psychological variables, optimism, future orientation, personal control and, symptoms reported by participants were entered as one set of predictors and social variables, relationship in family, opportunities for personal growth in family and system maintenance in family were entered as second set of predictors.

Satisfaction with Past Life as Predicted by Psychosocial Variables: Both in chronically ill and healthy group none of the psychological and social variables significantly predicted satisfaction with past life.

Satisfaction with Present Life as Predicted by Psychosocial Variables: Table 32 shows that in chronically ill group of participants satisfaction with present life was significantly predicted by three psychological variables, namely, future orientation, optimism and physical symptoms reported [F (l, 179) = 13.14, P<.000]. These three variables together explained 18.3 per cent of total variance in the criterion variable. Future orientation was the best predictor which explained 12.3 per cent of variance in the criterion variable, independently, followed by optimism which accounted for 3.9 per cent of total variance in the criterion variable, then comes physical symptoms reported which was found responsible for 2.1 per cent of variance in the criterion variable. Examination of the beta weights suggests that future orientation and optimism had positive contribution and physical symptoms reported had negative contribution in the prediction of criterion variable. Table 32 shows that in chronically ill group of participants satisfaction with present life was significantly and positively predicted by social variable, relationship in family [F (1, 179) = 17.08, P<.01] which accounted for 8.8 per cent variance in this criterion variable.

Satisfaction with Future Life as Predicted by Psychosocial Variables: Table 32 shows that in chronically ill group of participants satisfaction with future life was positively predicted by two predictors viz. personal control and, future orientation [F (1,179) = 75.15, P<.000]. These two predictors together explained 45.9 per cent of total variance in the criterion variable. Personal control was the best predictor which explained 41.6 per cent variance in the criterion variable independently, followed by future orientation, which accounted for 4.3 per cent variance in the criterion variable.

Table 32: Psychosocial Variables as Predictors of SWL in Different Time Zones

Psychological Variables					
Chronically ill Group					
Criterion = Present SWL					
Predictors	**R**	**R^2**	**R^2 Change**	**Beta**	**t**
Future Orientation	.35	.12	.123	.29	4.08**
Optimism	.40	.16	.021	.15	2.49**
Physical Symptoms Reported	.43	.18	.021	-.15	-2.14**
Criterion = Future SWL					
Personal Control	.65	.42	.416	.48	6.93**
Future Orientation	.68	.46	.043	.26	3.75**
Criterion = Total SWL					
Personal Control	.51	.20	.261	.38	4.83**
Future Orientation	.53	.29	.025	.20	2.49**
Healthy Group					
Criterion = Future SWL					
Personal Control	.63	.48	.479	.58	6.06**
Optimism	.76	.57	.091	.32	3.31**
Criterion = Total SWL					
Personal Control	.41	.17	.171	.41	3.31**
Social Variables					
Chronically Ill Group					
Relationship in Family	.30	.08	.088	.30	4.13**

Note: P<.01**

Table 32 presents that in healthy group of participants satisfaction with future life was positively predicted by two variables, namely, personal control and optimism [F(1,54) = 34.46, P<.000]. These two variables together explained 57.0 per cent of total variance in the criterion variable. Personal control was the best predictor which explained 47.9 per cent variance in the criterion variable independently, followed by optimism, which accounted for 9.1 per cent variance in the criterion variable.

Total Temporal Satisfaction with Life as Predicted by Psychosocial Variables: In chronically ill group of participants total temporal satisfaction with life was positively predicted by personal control and future orientation [F(1,179) = 35.433, P<.000] which together accounted for 28.6 per cent of total variance in the criterion variable. Personal control was the best predictor, which accounted for 26.1 per cent of total variance in the criterion variable independently, followed by future orientation which is responsible for 2.5 per cent of total variance in the criterion variable (Table 32).

Table 32 presents that in healthy group of participants total temporal satisfaction with life was significantly and positively predicted by personal control [F (1, 54) = 10.935, P<.002]. Personal control explained 17.1 per cent variance in the criterion variable.

Psychosocial Variables as Predictors of Total Temporal Satisfaction with Life in Different Patient Groups: In cancer patient group of participants personal control had significantly and positively predicted total temporal satisfaction with life [F(1,34) = 5.94, P<.000]. Personal control explained 20.3 per cent variance in the criterion variable (Table 33). In diabetic patient group of participants personal control significantly and positively predicted total temporal satisfaction with life [F (1, 54) = 16.58, P<.000]. Personal control explained 29.8 per cent variance in the criterion variable (Table 33). In heart patient group of participants future orientation significantly and positively predicted total temporal satisfaction with life [F (1, 54) = 21.36, P<.000]. Future orientation explained 28.7 per cent variance in the criterion variable (Table 33). In the group of patients afflicted with both diabetes and heart diseases personal control [F (1, 34) = 4.83, P<.000] significantly and positively predicted 38.1 per cent variance in the criterion variable.

Table 33 shows that in the group of patients afflicted with both diabetes and heart diseases system maintenance in family [F (1, 34) = 8.66, P<.000] significantly and negatively predicted total temporal satisfaction with life. It explained 20.8 per cent variance in the criterion variable.

Table 33: Psychosocial Variables as Predictors of SWL in Different Patient Groups

Psychological Variables						
Groups	**Predictors**	**R**	**R^2**	**R^2 Change**	**Beta**	**t**
Cancer Patients	Personal Control	.45	.20	.203	.45	2.90**
Diabetic Patients	Personal Control	.55	.29	.298	.55	4.73**
Heart Patients	Future Orientation	.54	.28	.287	.53	4.62**
Patients with both Diabetes and Heart	Personal Control	.62	.38	.381	.62	4.51**
Social Variables						
Patients with both Diabetes and Heart	System Mainte-nance in Family	.46	.20	.208	-.46	-2.94**

Note: P<.01**

SECTION-E

Content analysis of the open ended and free listing interview data have been presented in this section.

Benefit-finding from Chronically-ill Health Condition

Table 34 presents the benefits as perceived by chronically ill patients from their long-term ill-health condition and its frequencies. After the content analysis a total of 11 such benefits were found.

Table 34: Perceived Benefit Finding from Negative Situation by Chronically Ill Groups

Perceived Benefits	*Frequency (N = 180)*	%
Unexpected Family support	90	50
Emotional support	72	40
Closeness in Relationships	63	35
Familial Bonding	63	35
Better understanding of people	54	30
Better understanding of life	45	25
Making short-term plans	36	20
Change in health habits	30	16.66
Recognizing one's own potentials	27	15
Faith in God	20	11.11
Positive attitude towards people	18	10

Goals and Aspirations: The chronically ill group of patients were asked to depict some of their goals and aspirations which they want to achieve in coming future. Table 35 presents the goals and aspirations as said by patients along with the frequencies. The goals and aspirations as stated by patients were categorized into 10 such categories.

Table 35: Goals and Aspirations as stated by Chronically Ill Groups

Goals and Aspirations	*Frequency (N = 180)*	*%*
Improving/stabilizing economic condition	104	57.77
Finding/retaining/improving job or work (self or family member)	100	55.55
Health (self)	90	50.00
Personal Growth	86	47.77
Construction/consolidation of property	84	46.66
Courtship/marriage/children (self)	76	42.22
Family relations	52	28.88
Education	44	24.44
Care by family	30	16.66
Marriage of family member	22	12.22

Fears of Patients

Table 36 shows the categories and frequencies of fears of chronically ill patients about their future. A total of six such categories of fears were found in content analysis.

Table 36: Fears Perceived by Chronically Ill Groups

Fears	*Frequency (N = 180)*	*%*
Death will be bothersome/distressful	162	90.00
Problems for family due to disease	104	57.77
Future of Children	69	38.33
Loneliness	58	32.22
Accident	32	17.77
Theft/Robbery	14	7.7

Causes Attributed by Patients for their Disease

Table 37 presents the categories of causes attributed by chronically ill patients for their illness. A total of 12 reasons were attributed by patients for their illness. Amongst them some causes are internal or external and some are controllable or uncontrollable causes.

Table 37: Causes Attributed by Chronically Ill Groups for their Illness

Causes	*Frequency (N = 180)*	*%*
Mental tension	46	25.55
Do not know	35	19.44
Heredity	22	12.22
Good and rich food	18	10.00
God's will	15	8.33
Irregularity	15	8.33
Fate/Destiny	11	6.11
Lack of exercise	9	5.00
Obesity	7	3.88
No physical activity	6	3.33
Use of Tobacco	5	2.7
Circumstances	3	1.6
Lack of Knowledge	2	1.1

Discussion

The findings reported in the preceding chapter have been subjected to elaborate discussion with a view to present the results in an integrated, meaningful and coherent manner and to present possible explanations for the obtained results. Such an attempt made in the present chapter will also be helpful in bringing out the implications of the findings of research.

Relationship in Coping Strategies and Psychological Variables

Effective coping may involve in maintaining and protecting social relationship as well as solving problems. Review of the literature indicated that psychological factors, personality characteristics and behavioural style act as resources (Parkes, 1986; Taylor, 1989). These are called resources because they promote more vigorous and persistent efforts to overcome stress. Hobfall (1988) defined resources as "those objects, conditions, personal characteristics or energies that are valued by the individual or that serve as means for attainment of valued resources." They provide ego-strength or some wealth to a person "to fall back upon" when one is saddled with difficulties, in life (Carver *et al.*, 1989; Taylor *et al.*, 1992; Carpenter and Scott, 1992). In the present investigation it was hypothesized that psychological and social resources, like, future orientation, optimism, personal control, family environment will strengthen the use of more active problem focused coping and lesser use of maladaptive coping strategies. It was also thought that coping strategies which one uses can also influence the quality of one's life and judgment of satisfaction in life. It is also expected that the psychological characteristics and resources will influence a person's quality of life through the use of the coping mechanisms which a person favours.

How do five global coping strategies i.e. active coping, adaptive coping, maladaptive coping, acceptance coping and coping through humour relate with psychological characteristics and social resources are discussed below—

Active Coping Strategies

There are certain social psychological processes like, a sense of control, optimism and future oriented outlook along with a cohesive and healthy relationship in family and system maintenance in family which may enhance the use of active coping strategies in chronically ill individuals. Researchers suggest that people who hold positive belief about themselves, have higher degree of personal control and envisage a positive future are more likely to use active coping strategies, both at the anticipatory stage when stressful event have not yet occurred and when they are actually taking place (Aspinwell and Taylor, 1999).

A variety of dispositional factors which appear to be important in coping processes and which were studied earlier include, self-efficacy (Bandura, 1977), optimism (Scheier and Carver, 1985), hardiness (Kobassa, Maddi and Kahn 1982), sense of coherence (Antonovsky, 1987) and internal locus of control (Lefcourt, 1991), family support (Fondacaro and Moos, 1987). Studies in the area of health crisis showed that personal and social recourses maximize the persistent efforts to handle the critical situation. Optimists tend to use problem focused coping strategies, whereas, pessimists prefer emotion focused coping strategies such as denial and fatalism (Carver *et al.*, 1989; Taylor *et al.*, 1992). The ability to remain optimistic even unrealistically optimistic in the face of adversity (Reed *et al.*, 1994; Taylor *et al.*, 1992) and the ability to find meaning in adverse experiences appears to be physiologically protective (Bower *et al.*, 1998).

Results of the present investigation (Table 7) showed that psychological characteristics of future orientation, optimism and personal control and social factors, namely, relationship in family and system maintenance in family are significant predictors of active coping strategies in chronically ill group of participants.

The three psychological variables jointly and positively predicted 28 per cent variance in criterion variable of active coping with problems. Active coping strategies may be protective in, as much as, there is a large and growing literature indicating that avoidant coping is inferior to active coping while facing a broad range of stressors and that it represent risk factor for psychological distress (Felton, Revenson and Hinrichson, 1984; Holahan and Moos, 1986, 1987a). Billings and Moos (1985) found that use of active and problem focused coping and minimal use of avoidant coping were associated with fewer physical and psychological symptoms and that patients who coped with problem solving and affect regulation had less severe dysfunctions.

Findings of the studies of Reed, Taylor and Kemeny, (1993), Thompson *et al.* (1993), Helgeson (1992) suggest that perception of control is beneficial for people facing serious loss or trauma and it is associated with active coping and better health. Results of the present investigation contribute to effective functioning and make the patients able to confront directly with the problem.

In the present investigation personal control emerges as important predictor of use of active coping strategies, when there was a crisis in life. Christensen, Turner, Smith, Holmen and Gregary (1991), reported that patients adapt best to chronic illness when they use a highly active and vigilant style of coping and this was done only when things seem controllable, on the other hand, when the medical context or disease is less controllable, a less active style of coping may be associated with better adherence. It is apparent from a glance at Tables 7 and 8 that having personal control becomes very important for coping when one is facing life threatening diseases. On the other hand, in normal healthy people personal control is not a preferred resource and may even lead to behavioural disengagement. For the chronically ill person living and adjusting with daily routine is not an easy task, especially after an acute episode of illness. One has to cope with illness, treatment regimen, pain, discomfort, disfigurement, as well as, taking medicine, dietary restrictions, economic problems, problems with family members and carrying a task of living as a useful member of society and family. Then personal control can come in handy for active coping, planning and positive reinterpretation (Table 7). Along with personal control, positive future time perspective is very important for coping in active manner. Table 7 shows that two components of active coping, i.e., suppression of competing activities and restraint coping predicted by future orientation. Those patients who are able to suppress distracting things are more likely to think and plan about future. Agrawal, Tripathi and Srivastava (1984), stated that impulse control denotes ego strength and it is a positive quality which may help a person to reflect on all facts of a problem and come up with the correct solution rather than give a quick and wrong solution.

Besides these psychological resources, two dimensions of family environment, cohesive relationships in family and system maintenance in family are important predictors of active coping strategies in chronically ill group of participants (Table 9). It can be said that the patients find courage for facing the disease in active manner, one who has a cohesive, less conflicting, more expressive, more caring and unconditionally supportive family environment. Along with this every member in the family tried to follow the rules set for family and take his responsibility also make the patients feel less bothered about the organization in family and this in turn helps him to concentrate more on to fight actively with complications of the disease. Studies in the area of health and other context showed that social resources can elevate coping efforts by enhancing self-efficacy, as well as, by providing information and guidance (Thoits, 1986). People who have more social contacts and networks rely more on active coping such as positive reinterpretation and seeking guidance and support and less an avoidance coping especially emotional ventilation (Holahan and Moos, 1987; Moos, Brennan, Fondacare and Moos, 1990).

Psychological variables did not systematically predict use of specific coping strategies in normal healthy group of participants. Perhaps, it means that there is greater variability in coping reactions in healthy people and psychological characteristics may be instrumental in making a person more flexible so that he can choose a coping strategy according to the situation. Personal qualities or dispositions, like, future orientation, optimism, personal control and social factors, like, relationship and system maintenance in family appears to be resources which are utilized to develop combined active coping strategies to meet the contingencies arising due to health problems. On the other hand, in case of healthy persons, these resources did not predict the type of coping which are used by healthy people. It is possible that if the group of healthy respondents had been larger then some more relationships between coping strategies and psychological, personal and social resources could have emerged.

To get a clear picture of how these psychosocial variables act in adjustment with and management of each disease and to find the predictive power of each psychosocial variable in the use of particular coping strategy in different patient groups, the data was analyzed separately for each group. Cancer patients have been using the combined active coping strategies which are needed to cope with the burden of disease are predicted by two psychological characteristics, namely, personal control and future orientation (Table 11). In this group system maintenance in family also predicted active coping. It is, therefore, evident that active coping is directly sustained by personal control and future orientation and indirectly by social support and system maintenance in family.

The results of the present investigation confirm the widespread assumption that active problem focused coping might reduce the level stress. Active problem focused coping strategies, such as planful problem solving or positive reappraisal (Heim *et al.*, 1987) reduce the impact of threatening events during the early stages of cancer diagnosis. This may be because that actively following treatment, planning for future course of action brings relief and diminishes uncertainty. In the case of diabetic patients, again personal control emerges an important psychological characteristic (Table 11), which leads to the use of active coping strategies. Coping with diabetes is not an easy task because lower production of insulin or irregular production in itself is not so dangerous, but the bulk of complications which arise from it, like, neuropathy, retinopathy, amputation, non-healing ulcers etc. can cause serious damage. It is, therefore, essential to have a sense of control on things for diabetics as lead to direct control of situations, plan for contingency and directly act on it. It is very difficult for a diabetic patient to deal with all the above-mentioned complications and symptoms related with them hence, if one feels in control he may act to avoid complications. In heart patients group of participants also personal control emerged as the best predictor of active coping strategies along with symptoms reported by patients. People with inclination to report psychological complications and symptoms tend to use more passive, avoidant coping strategies (e.g. Turner and Clancy, 1986). Having a sense of control on the other hand, generally promotes strategies like, planning and realistically changing goals which are reachable (Thompson and Wierson, 2000). Perhaps, a sense of control makes the patients believe that although they are vulnerable to heart attacks but they can control it by using dietary charts, exercises and medicines. In heart patients group of participants active coping strategies was also predicted by relationship in family. Other empirical evidences suggest that personal control hastens the recovery from CHD and improves cardiac symptoms (Fontana, Kerns, Rosenberg and Colonese, 1989; Kulik and Mahler, 1993).

In patients afflicted with diabetes and heart problems, a future oriented outlook (Table 11) predicts active coping strategies. The reason may be that patients suffering from these two chronic and serious diseases have to deal with the complications related to both, simultaneously. In order to remain well adjusted and fully fledged in life, a futuristic outlook might work as a jack. Only in this group of patients social variable, personal growth in family was predicted active coping strategies. It suggests that if families of patients provide an opportunity for personal growth in the form of recreational activities and independence, it increases the likelihood of using active coping strategies by patients.

It can be concluded on the basis of above-mentioned findings that in all the participants of various patient groups separately, as well as, in the total patient group of participants suffering from different chronic illnesses, tendency to effectively and actively manage the chronic disease, is fostered by some psychological dispositions like, having sense of control, optimism and future oriented outlook along with supportive and caring family relationships and system in family.

Adaptive Coping Strategies

Adaptation means the psychological processes employed by the individual to manage environmental demands (Lazarus and Folkman, (1984a). Adaptive coping strategies were significantly predicted by two dimensions of family environment scale, namely, relationship in family and personal growth in family in healthy group of participants (Table 9). However, in chronically ill group of participants adaptive coping strategies were neither significantly predicted by social variables, nor by psychological variables.

Healthy individuals, who have supportive family members, committed to one another, express their feelings and thoughts openly, adapt more effectively to stressful situations. Along with this if family members independently make their own decisions and are working for their personal growth only then it becomes difficult to adopt to adverse condition, for healthy people. Religion, a component of adaptive coping strategies was negatively predicted by future orientation and personal control (Table 11). In COPE scale the items for use of religion as a coping strategy for the solution of problems shows excessive dependence on religion. Furthermore, one item is concerned with excessive praying. It is only understandable that if a patient feels that things are out of control, he starts depending on prayer only. Similarly, if a person depends excessively on prayer to make everything well, he may think that I pray and God will take care, I need not do anything and he may not plan for his own future at his own level, hence, those healthy people who have future oriented outlook do not depend on God for removing all their difficulties and do not excessively pray to him for this purpose. Similarly, instrumental social support, a component of adaptive coping, positively predicted by total symptoms reported in healthy group of participants. This suggests that those healthy participants who express more neurotic tendencies are likely to demand more instrumental social support (Table 12).

Adaptive coping strategies were preferred more by healthy group of participants than by chronically ill individuals. Actually, a coping style is determined by the interaction of personal needs and preferences and the constraints of the current situation. Pearlin and Schoolar (1978) suggested that whether specific coping strategies will prove to be effective or not depends on the type of stress encountered. This line of reasoning can explain the differences in the use of various coping strategies by healthy and chronically ill group of participants.

Maladaptive Coping Strategies

Evidences from numerous empirical studies suggested that maladaptive, avoidant coping behaviours may be responsible for causing, maintaining and even exacerbating physical ill health and threat to well-being also (e.g. Carver *et al.*, 1993; Suls and Fletcher,

1985). Findings of the present study show that psychological characteristics of optimism negatively predicted use of maladaptive coping strategies in chronically ill group of participants (Table 10). Optimism also significantly and negatively predicted two components of maladaptive coping strategies, behavioural disengagement and venting of emotions. Carver *et al.* (1993) also reported that optimists, as compared with pessimists tended to use the negative coping responses like disengagement. Table 11 also shows that coping strategy of mental disengagement was negatively predicted by personal control and the physical symptoms reported by chronically ill group of participants. It seems that those patients who perceive that they have their life under control also dwell less on physical symptoms, which they experience due to disease and they mentally disengage to lesser extent. The patient thinks he/she can control aspects of disease, as well as, his/her life, so it is not needed to disengage from his/her mind from his/her problems, by daydreaming or seeing movies etc. or sleeping.

A somewhat unprecedented result was found in the present investigation. One of the maladaptive coping strategies, denial was positively predicted by personal control in chronically ill group. Perhaps, denial has a positive value in chronic illness. One tries to act in a normal manner in an adverse situation by denying that disease has disabling effect, rather one says that disease is not disabling him/her. Gentry, Foster and Haney (1972) also reported that patients with myocardial infarction who deny their illness have less anxiety. Similarly, Levenson, Mishra, Hamer and Hastillo (1989) and Levine *et al.*, (1987) also reported that denial predicts better medical outcome during acute hospitalization for coronary artery heart disease. It was evident that avoidance coping strategies, such as denial and withdrawl, were associated with psychological distress (Holmes and Stevenson, 1990).

The results of multiple regression analyses for different patient groups, separately, revealed that amongst participants of cancer patient group reporting physical symptoms positively and significantly predicted use of maladaptive coping strategies. In cancer patient group of participants too social variable, personal growth in family (Table 9) predicted use of maladaptive coping strategies. This is understandable because personal growth dimension of this family environment scale refers to greater independence and freedom to pursue hobbies and recreational activities. In patients of chronic diseases, however, it is possible when they are giving this freedom they start misusing this facility and this, in turn, tend to engage them in more maladaptive coping strategies, like, mental and behavioural disengagement, denial and venting of emotions. On the other hand, relationship in the family (Table 9) predicts negatively and significantly the use of maladaptive coping strategies. The reason behind this finding is also very clear. Cohesive relationship within the family as strengthens forces against stress and dissuade the person to use maladaptive coping strategies.

In participants of heart patient group optimism negatively predicted the use of maladaptive coping strategies (Table 8). A number of other studies have also reported similar findings. For example: Long and Sangeter (1993) reported that optimists use problem solving coping and pessimists use wishful thinking, which predicts poor adjustment. Actually, optimism leads to constructive thinking and this constructive thinking, in turn, enables the person to act directly to solve the problem. In participants of heart patients group none of the social variables predicted maladaptive coping strategies but in the group of patients suffering from both diabetes and heart problems good relationship in family (Table 9) negatively predicted maladaptive coping. These findings show that supportive family members may act as buffers to minimize complexities arising due to combination of two chronic diseases at a time and provide support to the distressed patients to deal with his problems and thereby discourage maladaptive efforts to overcome the problems (Dakof and Taylor, 1990).

Although psychological and social variables systematically did not predict use of specific strategies in healthy group of participants, but it was found that reporting psychological symptoms (Table 8) predicted use of maladaptive coping strategies in this group. There is some evidence to suggest that neurotic preoccupation with the symptoms of distress is counter-productive and has adverse effect on adjustment. It is under stable, for example if a person reports and is bothered by headache, loss of sleep, anxiety, disappointment and a feeling that life is a burden, then, one is likely to stop coping actively with the problem and, retreat behind such maladaptive coping strategies as mental disengagement and venting of emotions. Present findings suggest such a course of thinking and acting.

Acceptance Coping

Acceptance of reality engages the person to reprioritize their goals. The individuals start to learn to live in their new situation. Acceptance is actually referred here as active acceptance. It means admitting that a problem exist or that an event happened and it cannot be changed. This acceptance orients the person towards constructive and developmental tasks. Findings of the present investigation show that system maintenance in family (Table 12) negatively predicted acceptance as coping strategy in patients. The reason may be that chronically ill patients, on the one hand, accepted the reality that it had happened to them, but there are certain family rules and regulations about daily routine activities. The illness of the patient sometimes restricts them to obey these rules or sometimes they feel they cannot do it due to illness. So, this reigned attitude tends to lesser use of acceptance as a coping strategy. In healthy group of participants acceptance not emerged as preferred coping strategy.

Humour Coping

Research evidences supported the view that humour or laughter and joking is a positive asset and stress moderator. Tables 11 and 12 show that use of humour as a coping strategy was significantly and negatively predicted by physical symptoms reported by chronically ill patient group of participants, whereas, in healthy group of participants, optimism was positively predicted humour coping strategy. These findings suggest that use of humour as a coping strategy decreases the likelihood of reporting more physical symptoms and, optimistic outlook increases the likelihood of using humour as a coping strategy in the wake of adversity in healthy group of participants. Perhaps, those who are healthy and not struck with any aversive stimulus at present, think positively that if there will be any such adverse condition, it would be beneficial to joke and laugh about it and in this way its intensity will be reduced. Rottan and Shats (1996) found that humour have utility as a pain reducer following orthopaedic surgery. Carver *et al.* (1993) have reported the ways of coping of early stage breast cancer patients in each of the five assessments at pre-surgery, post-surgery and then 3, 6, and 12 months follow-ups, use of humour was positively associated with optimism. The results of the present investigation suggest that for patients dwell obsessively on disease symptoms, they are unable to use humour for coping. Symptoms reporting were negatively predicted humour coping in patient group of participants also. In the case of cancer patient group of participants, perception of controllability increases the probability of using humour as a coping strategy.

Findings support the interpretation that these resources are important for prevention of disease. The findings of this investigation highlights the importance of the psychological resources in chronic illnesses. This information is important for clinical trials of various treatment methods and counselling sessions.

Relationship in Coping Strategies and Quality of Life and Life Satisfaction

The individuals coping abilities are found to have influence on overall health. These coping abilities are influenced by a number of psychological and social characteristics (Cohen *et al.* 1982). Findings of the present investigation as discussed previously also shares this view. It was hypothesized that coping styles are influenced by psychosocial factors, and at the same time, these particular coping styles play a role in determining a person's perception of his quality of life and satisfaction with life.

Total Quality of Life

Quality of life is concerned with perception of goals, expectations, experiences of individual in his socio-cultural context and the value system in which he lives. The greater use of active coping and lesser use of maladaptive coping strategies predicts increase in the rating of his/her total quality of life by the chronically ill group of participants (Table 15). Other researchers like Aldwin and Revenson (1987); Aspinwell and Taylor (1992) also found relationship between active coping and well-being. Active coping is preferred by most persons and is highly effective in stress reduction (Gal and Lazarus, 1975). The reason behind this may be that active coping provides a sense of mastery over the stressor, engagement in task oriented behaviour and discharge of energy following exposure to threat. By using more active and less maladaptive coping strategies the patient is able to modify the threat of stressor, maintain balance, plan for strategies to reduce the intensity of stress and all this leads him to evaluate his life as having good quality. These findings are also strengthened by the results shown in Table 16. This table shows that two components of combined active coping strategies, namely, active coping and suppression of competing activities significantly and positively predict better perception of quality of life in patients afflicted with chronic health problems. It seems that the more the patient directly confronts his problem, the better the rates his quality of life. Wagner, Armstrong and Laughlin (1995) also found similar results in their study on seriously ill cancer patients. More the patients suppressed competing activities to focus on the management of problem; the better they evaluated their quality of life. The results explain that not taking part in activities which might be disturbing would be associated with perceived quality of life.

When adaptive coping strategies were entered with other four global coping strategies in stepwise multiple regression analysis adaptive coping strategies did not predict total quality of life, but when components of adaptive coping strategies were entered separately, religion (Table 16) negatively predicted the total quality of life. This finding can be interpreted along with the findings described in the previous section that, greater sense of control reduces the probability of using religion as a coping strategy. More use of religious practices in order to make the problems go away decreases perception of quality of life as good in chronically ill group of participants. Problems don't go away simply because one prayed to God at the same time one does not engage in active coping to reduce the problems. This indicates that having a sense of control encourages actively tackling the problem and promotes lesser dependence on God for problem solving. This, in turn, helps the individual to perceive that quality of one's life is good. Two maladaptive coping strategies, namely, behavioural disengagement and venting of emotions negatively predicted quality of life in chronically ill group of participants (Table 16). These findings confirm that simply day dreaming or not thinking about the problem does not cure the problem; furthermore, since one is not doing much directly for the management of disease, the problems generated by disease accumulate. Focus on venting of emotions is a coping skill which based on absorption that interferes with problem solving. Mayou and Bryant (1987) reported that avoidance coping strategies are negatively correlated with subsequent quality of life.

In healthy group of participants, only one coping strategy, i.e. behavioural disengagement, a component of maladaptive coping strategies, negatively and significantly predict good quality of life. The reasons for this finding are the same as charted out above for chronically ill group of participants.

Physical Quality of Life

Physical quality of life (as measured by WHOQOL) includes the various dimensions related with physical functioning, like, unpleasant physical sensations and pain, level of energy and fatigue, sleep and rest, mobility, ability to perform usual daily living activities and a person's dependence on medication.

Results of this investigation shown in Table 18 indicate that two global coping strategies, namely, combined active coping and acceptance coping predict good physical quality of life. Along with these two components of combined active coping strategies, i.e. suppression of competing activities and planning also significantly predict physical quality of life in chronically ill group of participants. The patient who evaluate their physical quality of life positively are those who plan for it, involve their energy to manage the disease. Perception of being in a good physical health is not contradicting with having chronic disease. In spite of disease perception is fostered by the psychosocial characteristics they possesses, namely, perception that one has control, futurity, optimism, supportive and caring relationships.

Psychological Quality of Life

Psychological quality of life consists of feelings of happiness, contentment and joy and lesser feelings of guilt, sadness and despair, a person's perception and judgment about his thinking, learning, meaning and concentration, self-esteem, a person's view about his body image and appearance also formulate the psychological quality of one's life. Results suggest that psychological quality of life is positively predicted by suppression of competing activities, active coping and negatively predicted by religion, behavioural disengagement and venting of emotions (Table 18) in chronically ill group of participants. These results indicate that if patients can concentrate on task at hand without bothering about competing activities and, don't show much dependence on religion, nor do they ventilate their emotions, but face the problems in an active manner, then they psychologically also feel better and enjoy the life even in adversity. Because by coping actively they might be able to retain their sense of self-worth, that they can control events, have self-esteem and positive about their body image and can concentrate on problem. In healthy group of participants psychological quality of life was not significantly predicted by coping strategies.

Social Quality of Life

Social quality of life as assessed through WHOQOL refers to the extent to which one feels companionship and support, one's desire to form intimate relationships and availability of practical assistance from family and friends and expression and enjoyment with sexual activities. In chronically ill group of participants social quality of life was significantly and positively predicted by active coping (Table 18) and negatively predicted by religion, instrumental social support, venting of emotions and behavioural disengagement (Table 18). Those patients who perceive their social quality of life positively use active coping to solve the problem. Negative prediction of social quality of life by instrumental social support coping strategy signifies that in intimate social relationship with family and friends support, care and companionship is inherent in it and any kind of instrumentality might weaken this bonding and puts strain of relationships.

In healthy group of participants social quality of life was positively predicted by emotional social support (Table 18). The healthy group of participants are not facing any critical problem at present. If they face a problem they seek emotional support from their social network and it reduces the stress aroused by the problem since this normally happens infrequently, it has positive outcome. This, in turn, helps in perception of better social quality of life.

Environmental Quality of Life

The environmental quality of life as measured through WHOQOL explores the physical safety and security a person has, comfort of the place where a person lives, person's views about his financial resources, availability and quality of health and social services, person's opportunity and desire to learn new skills, person's ability, opportunity and inclination to participate in leisure activities, general aesthetic of physical environment and availability of transport services. Positive evaluation of this environmental quality in life is also predicted by active coping strategies in chronically ill patient group of participants. These findings can be interpreted in the light of results described in previous section that having a greater sense of control, positive expectation and future oriented outlook promotes the use of active coping strategies. Due to this tendency to act directly to do something increases the likelihood to evaluate the things that are present in the environment positively. Not only this chronically ill patient also feels that it don't make a change in physical environment according to the regimen of my disease, it would become difficult to handle the disease properly.

In healthy group of participants humour (Table 18) predicted good environmental quality of life. The healthy individuals laugh and joke on the physical environment and do not feel bad about the deprivation.

General Health Quality of Life

General health quality of life examines the ways in which people assess their overall quality of life, health and well-being. Results suggest that this assessment is influenced by how people plan to focus on management of disease and restrain themselves. This planning and restraining enhances general health quality of life. Lesser use of maladaptive coping and mental disengagement (Table 18) also promotes general health quality of life.

Life Satisfaction

Life satisfaction is an important aspect of personality and overall adjustment. It is a cognitive judgmental process. It was hypothesized in the present investigation that this cognitive judgment is influenced by psychosocial factors on the one hand and the type of coping strategies used by the individuals on the other hand. In this sub-section firstly the results of the total temporal satisfaction with life as related with coping strategies is discussed and then the three temporal aspects, namely, past, present and future satisfaction is also discussed.

Total Temporal Satisfaction with Life

Judgment of satisfaction with life as a whole is influenced by the types of coping strategies used. Combined active coping strategies (Table 19) were found to be effective in promoting the level of satisfaction. Throughout the findings of the present investigation reported that active coping strategies are important for well-being. It does not mean that active coping strategies resolve all the problems, suffering and complaints faced by the chronically ill patients, but it does mean that combined active coping strategies contribute in realistic acknowledgement of problems and provide effective ways of coping with it. Certain psychosocial characteristics, like, optimism, future orientation and personal control promote and maintain positive overall satisfaction with life (e.g., Lewinshon, Render and Seely, 1991). Judgment of satisfaction is a cognitive process and it seems logical that only laughing on the situation may not reduce the stress induced by it. Therefore, this type of coping strategy may not allow a person to evaluate his life satisfactory. Although Carver *et al.* (1993) reported that use of humour have beneficial prospective effects on the subjective well-being. But in the long run humour coping strategy would not be beneficial because a chronically ill patient has to fight with the disease and maintain a good quality of life.

When the predictive pattern of five global coping strategies in different patient groups were considered, again, it was found that in three patient groups, namely, cancer patients, diabetic patients and heart patients judgment of satisfaction in life is predicted by the use of active coping strategies (Table 20).

Only in the group of patients suffering from both diabetes and heart problems adaptive coping strategies predicted satisfaction with life (Table 21). This may be that in this group of patients the complications related to both of the diseases make them more vulnerable to severe and recurring attacks of complications, so they need more emotional, as well as, instrumental social support, which characterize adaptive coping.

Satisfaction with Past Life

Life satisfaction as a whole is evaluated on the basis of past experiences, present situations and future expectations. Satisfaction with past life is not predicted by coping. The past had gone, therefore, active, adaptive or maladaptive coping strategies of present cannot do anything to change or modify the past experiences. Only humour coping significantly and negatively predicted satisfaction with past life (Table 19). However, laughing at past make people more dissatisfied with their past.

Satisfaction with Present Life

Satisfaction with present life is predicted by combined active coping strategies, as well as, three components of it, namely, active coping, restraint coping and positive reinterpretation coping strategies in chronically ill group of participants (Table 19). The patients have to manage their treatment regimen dietary charts, exercise schedules, meetings with doctors etc., in the present, therefore, it is very necessary for them to act, plan and work directly. This confrontative, problem focused coping strategy, in turn, tends to assess present life as satisfactory.

Satisfaction with Future Life

Satisfaction with future life is somehow influenced by the satisfaction with present life. Results show that satisfaction with future life was also predicted by combined active coping strategies and adaptive coping strategies in chronically ill group of participants (Table 19). These findings can be explained in the light of earlier findings of this investigation as presented in previous pages. Those who actively cope in present life and assess it satisfactory also feel that they can continue this style of coping and see their future life will also be satisfactory. As active coping strategies was predicted by future oriented and optimistic outlook, as well as, satisfaction with future life is also predicted by future orientation.

In healthy group of participants only one coping strategy i.e. venting of emotions predicted satisfaction with future life. This is a strange finding and only a post hoc guess can be hazarded. Number of participants in healthy group was less, so one cannot totally rely on this finding. Since in this group all coping strategies were employed and none was favoured, it is apparent that if healthy people are able to express and ventilate their emotions in present time they evaluate their life in future as satisfactory.

In nutshell findings suggest that combined active coping strategies are effective coping strategies to deal with problems faced by patients suffering from chronic diseases and these strategies help the patients to feel and describe their lives as full of quality in all domains and satisfactory at present and in future.

Relationship in Psychosocial Variables, Quality of Life and Life Satisfaction

When people find themselves in difficult situations like, suffering from a chronic disease, they often strive to actively minimize its negative impact (Taylor 1983, 1989). Results of the present investigation as discussed in the previous sections also provide supportive evidence. When people hold positive expectations regarding their abilities to deal with hardships, they cope effectively with it, therefore, this positive belief is associated with positive outcomes and well-being (Snyder *et al.*, 1991; Taylor, 1983, 1989). Psychosocial factors, affect the choice of coping strategies on the one hand and perception of quality of life and satisfaction with life on the other. How do these psychosocial variables influences the well-being has been discussed below.

Total Quality of Life

Personal control and optimism (Table 26) predicted accounted for better evaluation of quality of life in chronically ill group of participants. Both personal control and optimism also predicted use of active coping strategies on the one hand and on the other hand the use of active coping strategies also predicted total quality of life. Both of these psychological characteristics of personal control and optimism affected quality of life directly also. It is logical that problem focused, direct, and active coping strategies which are geared towards planning and modifying some aspects of the stressful situation are associated with more positive outcomes when the encounter is perceived as controllable (Folkman, 1984). Patients adapt best to chronic illness when they use highly active style of coping for medical context which allows greater patient control (Christenson, Turner, Smith, Holman and Gregory, 1991). Along with controllability, optimism was also found important for well-being. It was also reported by other researches that tendency to look at brighter side is associated with better mood, more perseverance and experience of better physical health (Peterson, 2000) and general well-being (Sweetman, Munz and Wheder, 1993). Furthermore, relationships in family and system maintenance in family also predict variance in total quality of life. These findings can also be interpreted in the light of the results discussed earlier that these two variables were best predictors of active coping strategies, as well as, quality of life. Patients with better relationship with family and friends are likely to rely on positive reinterpretation, planning, support seeking and care given by them and this, in turn, makes them perceive quality in life. Caring and supportive relationship also predicted quality of life in healthy group of participants.

Although those people who are healthy and are not facing any serious problem at present, even then in their normal course of life they need care, support, emotional expression, cohesiveness in their families. This strong family bonding makes them inclined to perceive their lives as having good quality in most respects. Findings of the present investigation are consistent with the psychological literature that shows benefits of positive beliefs about personal control and optimism.

These results show that these psychological characteristics have both direct and indirect influence on one's behaviour. These characteristics have been seen to predict variance in the usage of active coping techniques, which in turn, promote satisfaction with life and perception that overall one has good quality of life. These psychological resources and good family relations and social relations also directly predicted better quality of life.

Physical Quality of Life

Physical quality of life is constituted by level of physical energy, proper sleep and rest, dependence on medication and overall physical functioning of the individual. Interesting to note that optimism (Table 26) predicted physical quality of life in chronically ill group of participants. A positive expectation that despite the serious life threatening health condition, I am physically active, not overtly dependent on medication and would be physically functional in future also leads to enhanced physical quality of life. Actually, optimism increases the level of confidence of individual, which, in turn, make them able to overcome pain and discomfort associated with disease and helps one to remain functional at physical level. In contrast to this those who are not afflicted with any serious disease may also be discouraged, complaining of psychological symptoms like problems in sleeping, fatigue, nightmares etc. These neurotic tendencies may produce the negative assessment of physical quality in life. The results show that psychological symptoms reporting were negatively predicting physical quality of life in healthy group of participants.

System maintenance in family (Table 27) also predicted physical quality of life in chronically ill group of participants. Every family has certain norms and rules about food, sleep, rest, recreation, outdoor activities and daily routine etc. Maintenance of these rules is dependent upon the level of commitment of family members. It appears that if a person is afflicted with a serious illness but one is expected to abide by family rules and commitment make them physically active and working. Along with system maintenance, the optimistic outlook of the patient encourages regularity and concern about physical functioning in future also.

Psychological Quality of Life

Encountering positive feelings, maintenance of self-esteem, positive about body image, all these formulate the psychological quality of life. Findings show that having a sense of control and optimistic outlook (Table 26) in chronically ill patients make them perceive psychological quality in their lives. It seems logical that control related beliefs along with positive expectancy give strength to the patient not to dwell negatively but try and healthy group of participants' relationship in family positively and significantly predicted variation in this criterion variable.

It may be that perhaps densely populated cities, like Gorakhpur, where basic infrastructure is overburdened, the inhabitants are not satisfied with environmental quality. They think that their personal strength and resources can do nothing to improve it. They, therefore, lean to their family for seeking support and care. This makes them perceive environmental quality as somewhat better, because family support in small cities compensate for infrastructural facilities available in cosmopolitan cities.

Social Quality of Life

Social quality of life refers to personal and social relationships and sexual expressivity. Those patients who had good personal and social relationships with family, friends and other important fellows in their lives and also they do not have sexual inhibitions, were not intended to report more physical complaints (Table 26) and this, in turn, increases the likelihood of perceiving better social quality of life. This is true for the healthy group of participants also, as relationships in family (Table 27) also predicted good social quality of life in this group of participants.

Environmental Quality of Life

The environmental quality of life is basically related with the facility of transportation, physical safety and security, hygiene etc. Surprisingly, none of the psychological variables had emerged as significant predictor of it. Both in chronically ill and chronically ill people to cope and also have satisfaction in future and also promote total satisfaction in healthy group.

Psychological characteristics of personal control optimism and future orientation predicted both quality of life and satisfaction with life. These psychological qualities construct better of quality in life and this perception helps me to adjudge one's present and future life as satisfactory.

General Health Quality of Life

This measure of general health quality of life is concerned with the overall satisfaction of individuals with their health and life as a whole. Personal Control and future orientation (Table 26) along with relationship in family and personal growth (Table 27) predicted general health quality of life amongst participants of chronically ill patients group. It was discussed in earlier sections also that a strong sense of control and positive futuristic look reinforces the belief of patients that he can modify, change or retain at least some aspects of his life even in adverse situations. If he has good cohesive family relations then this sense become even strong. The motivational value related with future time perspective helps the patients to engage in health enhancing behaviours also (e.g. Lennings, 2000; Lang and Carstensen, 2002).

It is apparent from the findings of the regression analysis for relationship between quality of life and psychosocial variables that self-regularity mechanisms, like, control beliefs, positive expectations about outcome, planning of distant future and supportive relationships help in maintaining and recovering levels of global, as well as, domain specific well-being (e.g., Brandstandter, 1998; Heckhausen, 1999; Taylor and Armor, 1996; Tesser and Martin,1996).

These findings further suggest that subjective feelings of chronically ill or healthy person—about his quality of life is very important in coping with critical extents. Psychological characteristics, like, sense of control, optimism, future time perspective and relationship and system in family foster the individual to assess quality of his life in all respects, through directly confronting with the problems and not to escape from it.

Life Satisfaction

Satisfaction with life reflects individuals' cognitive judgment of situation of their own lives as a whole. Researchers of working on subjective well-being are trying to discover how an individual summarizes his life as a whole. An individual may use both situational induced and salient information and personality dispositions (Suh and Diener, 1999) to construct his judgment on his life satisfaction. Certain psychological characteristics, such as, hope (Snyder *et al.*, 1991), optimism (e.g., Scheier and Carver, 1993) and expectancy for control (Grob, *et al.*, 1999) appear to influence subjective well-being judgment. Results of the present study also show that sense of controllability and future orientation (Table 32) are significant predictors of total temporal satisfaction with life in chronically ill group of participants. Personal control also emerge as significant predictor of total temporal satisfaction with life in healthy group of participants. It appears that, perceived control rather the actual control is the key to psychological well-being (Abranson *et al.*, 1978; Bandura, 1977). Amongst participants suffering from chronic illness personal control and futurity appear to become much more important, because the control related beliefs and future oriented outlook helps the individual to find a meaningful life ahead even in adverse circumstances.

These positive attitudes are important as they allow the person to prepare for future stresses, like, rigorous treatment regimen, acute episodes of illness, or economic burden imposed by disease etc., and ensure that the situation will not become intolerable (Miller, 1979). These results clearly show that being afflicted with any threatening diseases does not shadow the life of the patients, if the patient still thinks and plans about future and perceives control over his or her life.

In healthy group of participants, because of the psychological symptoms (Table 32), they are trying to reinterpret their conditions but this is not improving their quality of life. These psychological variables are not influencing their quality of life directly. They are influencing their satisfaction with life, future and present satisfaction with life. Sometimes, some psychological variables have different influences on adoption of coping strategies and satisfaction with life. For example, psychological symptoms reporting has been found to predict use of positive reinterpretation, whereas, having personal control may predict behavioural disengagement in healthy group. Nevertheless, behavioural disengagement predicts lesser temporal satisfaction and perception of quality of life in healthy group of participants. On the other hand, personal control and future orientation predict higher satisfaction with future life (Table 32). It appears that having greater personal control in life can inspire them to feel that they will have a satisfaction future life, but if one has this tendency and encounters problems sometimes, one may disengage oneself behaviourally from the activity, when he does not succeed. This maladaptive coping tendency to quit things that one does not succeed has a dampening effect on perception of quality of life. It is, therefore, apparent that adoption of various techniques of coping is more variable in participants of healthy group.

Satisfaction with Present Life

Assessment of life satisfaction is dependent upon how much an individual is satisfied with his present life. As far as, satisfaction with present life is concerned, future orientation, optimism, reporting of physical symptoms and relationship in family (Table 32) emerged as significant predictors of satisfaction with present life in chronically ill group of participants. These participants were afflicted with such diseases which were disrupting their life in many respects. Thinking and planning about future and optimistic outlook make them satisfied even in present adverse conditions. Along with these psychological characteristics the family support is also very important. Cohesiveness, less conflict and more expressive environment within family, also gives some amount of relief and satisfaction. These positive factors help the patient not to bother about his physical pain and discomforts him evaluate his present life satisfactory.

Satisfaction with Future Life

Results show that personal control and future orientation in chronically ill group and personal control and optimism in healthy group of participants significantly predicted satisfaction with future life.

From the review of literature it is apparent that controllability enhances the level of confidence and future oriented outlook presents a vision which motivates the individual to pursue his goals. Optimistic outlook is awaited. It appears that in order for an individual to be satisfied in future, one needs to have a sense of control at present and an extended future time perspective. Both of these qualities helps the individual to fight with health calamities, as well as, other serious problems of life, and prepare the individual to be a well adjusted person in future who is satisfied and happy.

Results of the present investigation demonstrated that personal control is very important in coping and it does influence satisfaction with life also. Personal control helps restore self-concept and self-esteem. This psychological functioning is also influenced by the kind of support and care given by the family of patient and by the system maintenance in family. These psychosocial characteristics of the patients, as well as, the family of patients ensure the psychological adjustment and well-being of them.

Interpretation of Qualitative Data

These psychosocial resources influence the use of particular coping strategies for ill people who are fighting chronic illness. Coping styles determine to a large extent whether a person succeeds or fails in dealing with stress. This success or failure leads to better or adverse physiological and behavioural responses that have consequences for health and well-being. These relationships can be uncovered through qualitative methods, as well as, quantitative methods. In the present investigation besides using standardized scales and measures, the researches also interviewed patients. Their responses were content analyzed. This open ended interview was based on four types of questions. These are: (i) Do you perceive that this long-term illness has resulted in something positive? Like what?, (ii) What your goals and aspirations are (iii) What are your fears?, (iv) What are the causes which you think are responsible for your illness? These questions were asked from patient participants only.

Benefits Finding from Negative Situation

Psychologists have tried to investigate whether victims perceive any benefits or gains from traumatic conditions and other medical problems (Affleck, Tennen, Rowe and Higgins, 1990; Tennen, Affleck, Urrows, Higgins and Mendola, 1992). Research evidences from heart attack survivors (Affleck, Tennen, Croog and Levine, 1987); women with breast cancer (Taylor, Lichtman and Wood, 1984); mothers of children with insulin-dependent diabetes (Affleck, Allen, Tennen, McGrade and Ratzen, 1985) and many others established the fact that ability to detect personal gains from threatening experiences may enhance psychological and physical well-being.

In the present investigation the patients afflicted with chronic health problems perceive gains from their life threatening traumatic experiences. Amongst the benefits which were named by patients were unexpected family support, emotional support, closeness in relations and familial relatedness were concerned with social resources. The reason is that such large number of people suffering from chronic illness perceive that when people are stricken with such life threatening conditions they have a new realization of their interdependence, they feel it is impossible for them to handle these conditions all alone people seek social support and start paying attention to the kind of support they were getting from others and how valued this was for them. These social resources and close relationships are perceived as gains resulting from adversity. The quantitative measures used in the present investigation and already discussed showed that relationships in family were an important predictor of active coping, as well as, perception of good quality of life. The quantitative analysis clarifies that good relationships within family in a crisis strengthen to the patient if one perceives them resources.

Importance of perception of social support is highlighted by the qualitative analysis. Weiner's attribution model emphasise that causal appraiser of an event determine the directions and magnitude of felt emotion due to that event. Some emotions are outcome dependent, like, general affective reaction, on the other hand, pride, anger or gratitude follows the causal attributions which are held responsible for an event. When a pleasant outcome is attributed to gratitude is elicited (Overwall *et al.*, 1995). It is the contention of the present researcher that perception that other family members are great resources generates the feeling of gratitude. Gratitude is a compound of admiration and joy. Functionally gratitude motivate the person to regard others, pro-social behaviour (McCullough, Kelpatrick, Emmons and Larson, 2001). They posited that gratitude typically results from and stimulates moral behaviours. There is now evidence to show that those people who consistently felt thankful and maintained gratitude logs scored higher on measures of psychological well-being and were also more likely to help others in need (McCollough and Witviliet, 2002), which generally improves life within a family. Reminding oneself to feel grateful has been listed as helpful coping behaviour. A greater sense of appreciation for life has been noted as a common positive reaction to major medical problems (Affleck and Tennen, 1996). Virtues are required excellence, gratitude is one such virtue and strangely a calamity like, and life threatening illness may be source through which this virtue is cultivated.

The other benefits as stated by chronically ill patients generally pertain to psychological growth. As 30 per cent and 25 per cent patients perceive that their illness benefited them in understanding people and life, respectively. Besides these a number of other valued lessons had been thought by illness, like, making short-term plans, changing health habits for the better, positive attitude etc. The patients had learned to make short-term plans, because they thought that the physical restrictions imposed by illness made it difficult to plan for and stick to long-term goals. Furthermore, success in attaining short-term plans give them a feeling of achievement and this, in turn, motivated them to plan for next goal.

Results also show that the lifestyle of the patients changed after the onset of chronic disease. There may be some health behaviour and habits, for example, smoking or overeating or late night sleeping, lack of exercise etc. which had been changed. Perceiving the advantages as arising from negative situations has adaption value. Rothbaum *et al.* (1982) suggested that discovery of positive meaning in adversity is a type of secondary control appraisal.

Goals and Aspirations

People pursue multiple goals in their life. Locke (1996) in their goal theory identified that goals determine the direction, intensity and duration of action. Sometimes people have to face situations, they have never experiences, such circumstances endure for prolonged periods like, a chronic illness they compel the individual to reprioritize or sometimes even curtail his goals and aspirations.

In present investigation patients were asked to list their goals for which they aspire. More than 50 per cent patients stated that they were working towards improvement in economic conditions some job for family members and of course, improvement in their own health condition. It is understandable that these people are suffering from life threatening diseases and the treatment of these diseases is very costly. So, they were aspiring to meet the increased needs of money and uplift their economic condition either by getting a better job, or work for themselves, or for a significant family member like, son. Another goal mentioned by patients was adopting better health habits and taking care of their health. The chronic diseases like cancer, or diabetes or heart problems force the victim to compromise on several fronts in their lives. These patients are generally very worried about their health. They, therefore, set a goal for them to improve health conditions within the limitations imposed by disease. It was already discussed in the last section that personal control, optimism, future orientation were related with effective coping as well as, with well-being. Researchers are agreed that progression towards goal is an important source of perceived control and general well-being (e.g. Emmons, 1986 Little, 1989). People who have important goals tend to be more energetic, experience more positive emotions and feel that life is meaningful (McGregor and Little, 1989).

A rather surprising result was found that 28.88 per cent patient aspire for improving and maintaining family relation. These patients on the one hand, perceived that family bonding and closeness in relationship increased after the diagnosis of the disease, they feel it should be improved even more, on the other hand. Perhaps, their illness restricted them in many respects and this stimulated need of belongingness in them. They also aspire for more care by family. Again limited physical functioning and mobility and other illness related restrictions make them aspire for more care. Although they thought that illness had tend them to perceive that family is giving all kinds of support to them but due to their own limitations and the fear that these limitations may increase in future, they may need more care and support from family.

Fears

Fear is an emotional response to physical threat or anxiety to uncertain stimuli. Fear is characterized as negative emotions. Many theoretical models assign that emotions are associated with specific action tendencies (Lazarus, 1991; Ottley and Jenkins, 1996; Tooby and Cosmides, 1990). Although chronically ill participants use active coping strategies to overcome negativity aroused by prolonged stress due to disease, they also value controllability, optimism and futurity, still they have some fears. Perhaps these fears are because of the life threatening nature of their disease. Cancer, diabetes and heart diseases are particularly dangerous because of their unpredictable course of progression. Everything may be normal but suddenly an episode of complications may occur. These uncertainties of disease instigate fear in the patients that their death may be troublesome. Besides the fear of anguish of death, patients have also panic that their disease may create problems for their loved ones. These diseases cause problems at many fronts like, financial crises, frequent hospitalizations, disability in working, loss of energy, problems for caregiver etc. Patients are also very concerned with the future of their children. Although being parents people are usually concerned with the future of their offspring, however, in the case of people afflicted with a life threatening disease which has unpredictable course, this concern has taken the shape of fear. Chronic illness put limits on the physical activities and mobility of the person and also restricts the social interactions to some extent. Perhaps, this is the reason that many patients have expressed the fear of loneliness.

Causal Attribution for Disease

Causal attributions are the explanations the victims provide for their own behaviour, as well as, for the actions of the others. Many researchers are agree that while facing chronic illness or disability, people commonly search the cause of their suffering (Taylor, 1983). These identified causes enhance coping by preserving the individual's sense of being in control (Higgins and Synder, 1991). Patients had listed the causes that were in their control, or even the causes which were not in their control. Controllable causes were mental tension, good and rich food, irregularity, lack of exercise, obesity, no physical activity, use of tobacco, and lack of knowledge. The uncontrollable causes were heredity, God's will and fate or destiny. Many a patients also stated that they don't know the cause but their doctor better know.

Conclusion

The psychological characteristics like personal control, optimism, and future orientation and social variables like, relationship in family act as moderator variable in stress, coping and well-being relationship. Moderator variables are those variables which control and potentially affect the strength of the relationship in independent and dependent variables. They moderate the effect of stress on perceived quality of life and satisfaction with life. Stress may be caused by daily hassles in case of healthy people, and life threatening events in the case of chronically ill people. The psychosocial variables like, personal control, future orientation, optimism and family relations moderate the effect of stress, through the appraisal of the situations. When a person learns that he has developed a life threatening and long lasting illness, he may become dejected and may think that his life is over, or he may remain optimistic and arguing that with new advancements in medicine, he will be able to conquer his disease. Optimism thus may or may not affect the course of his illness but it is bound to affect his well-being, satisfaction and happiness. The findings of this investigation showcase that this is what actual happening is.

Personal control, optimism and having future goals render meaning to life, which is conducive to perception of good quality of life, satisfaction and well-being. Coping strategies which one employs, especially in the case of chronic illness, act as mediating variables. By definition mediating variables are explanatory constructs which account for the relationship between predictor and a criterion variable. Use of more active coping by chronically ill patients, for example, yielded a feeling in the patient that he can still control the situation, thus enhancing the satisfaction. This exemplifies how personal control may moderates the effect of perceived stress by chronic illness on one's well-being.

The prevalence of lifestyle diseases in India makes it pertinent to study the behavioural and lifestyle variables, which can alter or prevent people from balling prey to these diseases and cater them better life. Based on these empirical findings it may be recommended to chronically ill patients to think positively, see a light of hope even in darkness and develop a belief that one has control over internal resources. A psychologist may help and give counselling to the patients to ripen such resources. This counselling, in turn, may help them to cope with disadvantageous circumstances effectively.

References

Abbey, A., Abramis, D.J. and Caplan, R. (1985). Effects of different sources on emotional well-being. *Basic and Applied Social Psychology*, 6, 111-129.

Abbey, A. and Andrews, F.M. (1985). Modelling the psychological determinants of life quality. *Social Indicators Research*, 16, 1-34.

Abel, Millicent H. (1998). Interaction of humour and gender in moderating relationships between stress and outcomes. *The Journal of Psychology*, 132, 267-276.

Affleck, G., and Tennen, H. (1996). Construing benefits from adversity: Adaptational significance and dispositional underpinnings. *Journal of Personality*, 64, 899-922.

Affleck, G., Tennen, H., Croog, S., and Levine, S. (1987). Causal attribution, perceived control and recovery from a heart attack. *Journal of Social and Clinical Psychology*, 5, 339-355.

Affleck, G., Tennen, H., Pfeiffer, C., and Fifield, C. (1987). Appraisals of control and predictability in adapting to a chronic disease. *Journal of Personality and Social Psychology*, 53, 273-279.

Agarwal, A. (2003). Future goals and life satisfaction. *Psychological Studies*, 48(1), 47-55.

Agarwal, A. and Pandey, A. (1998). Coping with chronic disease: Role of Psychosocial variables. *Psychological Studies*, 43 (1 and 2), 58-64.

Agarwal, A. and Srivastava, M. (1981). Significance of time perspective in reflection impulsivity. *Psychological Studies*, 26, 100-103.

Agarwal, A. and Srivastava, M. and Tiwari, S. (1984). Development of time perspective: Its relation with conceptual and temporal judgment. Paper presented at U.G.C. National Seminar on Child Development, NCERT, New Delhi.

Agarwal, A. and Tiwari, S. (1988). Future Orientation: A mediator in temporal coding. *International Journal of Psychology*, 23, 151-163.

Agarwal, A. and Tripathi, I. (2000). Chronic illness, symptoms and efficacy in children as related to some psychological characteristics of mothers. *Psychology and Developing Societies*, 12(1), 31-42.

Agarwal, A. and Tripathi, K.K. (1984). Influence of prolonged deprivation, age and culture on the development of future orientation. *European Journal of Social Psychology*, 14, 451-453.

Agarwal, A., Tripathi, K.K. and Srivastava, M. (1983). Psychological implications of time perspective. *International Journal of Psychology*, 18, 367-380.

Agarwal, A. and Tripathi, L.B. (1979). Time perspective: II development and empirical validation of a new tool. *Psychological Studies*, 24, 59-65.

Akinci, F., Yildirim, A., Gozu, H., Sargin, H., Orbay, E., and Sargin, M. (2008). Assessment of health related QOL (HRQOL) of patients with type 2 diabetes in Turkey. *Diabetes Research Clinical Practice*, 79, 117-123.

Aldwin, C., Fellowmen, S., Scheeta, C., Coyne, J.I. and Lazarus, R. (1980). *Ways of Coping Checklist: A process measure*. Paper presented at the American Psychological Association's Annual Conference, Montreal, Canada.

Aldwin, C. and Revenson, T.A. (1987). Does coping help? A reexamination of the relation between coping and mental health. *Journal of Personality and Social Psychology*, 53, 337-348.

Anand, K. (2000). *Report on assessment of burden of major non-communicable disease in India*. World Health Organization, New Delhi.

Andrews, F.M. and Withey, S.B. (1976). *Social Indicators of Well-being: America's perception of life quality*. New York: Plenum.

Antonovsky, A. (1987). *Unravelling the Mystery of Health*, San Francisco: Jassey-Bass.

Appeals, A. and Mulder, P. (1989). Fatigue and heart disease: The association between "Vital exhaustion" and past, present and future coronary heart disease. *Journal of Psychosomatic Research*, 33, 727-738.

Appeals, A. and Otten, F. (1992). Exhaustion as precursor of cardiac death. *British Journal of Clinical Psychology*, 31, 351-356.

Argyle, M. (1987). *The Psychology of Happiness*. London, England: Methuen.

Aspinwell, L.G. and Taylor, S.E. (1992). Modelling cognitive adaptation: A longitudinal investigation of the impact of individual differences and coping on college adjustment and performance. *Journal of Personality and Social Psychology*, 63, 989-1003.

Aspinwell, L.G. and Taylor, S.E. (1997). A stitch in time: Self regulation and proactive coping. *Psychological Bulletin*, 121, 417-436.

Auerbach, A.M. (1989). Stress management and coping research in the health care setting: An overview and methodological commentary. *Journal of Consulting and Clinical Psychology*, 57, 388-395.

Baca, D.P., George, S.M.L. and Albertson Owens, S.A. (1999). *Coping and life satisfaction in younger and older adults*. Poster session presented at the meeting of the Geronotological Society of Aging Conference. San Francisco, C.A.

Bahnson, C.B. (1981). *Stress and cancer: The state of the art*. Psychosomatic, 22, 207-220.

Balfour, L., White, D.R., Schiffrin, A., Dougherty, G. and Dufresne, J. (1993). Dietary disinhibition, perceived stress and glucose control in young Type I diabetic women. *Health Psychology*, 12, 33-38.

Band, E.B. (1990). Children's coping with diabetes: Understanding the role of cognitive development. *Journal of Pediatric Psychology*, 15, 27-41.

Bandura, A. (1977). Self-Efficacy: Towards a unifying theory of behavioural change. *Psychological Review*, 84, 191-215.

Bar-On, D. (1986). Professional models vs. patient model in rehabilitation after heart attack. *Human Relations*, 39, 917-932.

Bar-On, D. (1987). Causal attribution and rehabilitation of myocardial infraction victims. *Journal of Social and Clinical Psychology*, 5, 114-122.

Basu, R. and Neogi, S. (1990). Association of coronary prove behaviour with coronary heart disease: A hospital based study. *Indian Journal of Psychological Issues*, 7(1), 14-19.

Basu, R. and Saha, M. (1985). Application of Jenkins Activity Survey (JAS) to identify the coronary prone behaviour pattern (Type A) in our domestic population. *Indian Journal of Clinical Psychology*, 11, 23-27.

Benson, S., Hahn, S., Tan, S., Janssen, O.E., Schedlowski, M., and Elsenbrush, S. (2010). Maladaptive coping with Illness in women with polycystic ovary syndrome. *Journal of Obstetric and Gynecologic and Neonatal Nursing*, 39(1), 40-45.

Berkman, L.F. (1985). The relationship of social network and social support to morbidity and mortality. In S. Cohen and S.L. Syme (Eds.) *Social Support and Health* (pp. 241-262), San Francisco: Academic Press.

Berkman L.F. (1995). *The role of social relations in health promotion.* Psychosomatic Medicine, 57: 245-54.

Bhatia, H. and Chadha, N.K. (1993). *Family Environment Scale.* Lucknow: Ankur Psychological Agency.

Bhatia, M.S., Tiwari, A., Balkrishna, S. and Gupta, H. (1990). Type A behaviour, life events and myocardial infraction. *Indian Journal of Medical Research*, 2, 95-100.

Bilge, F. and Saltuk, S. (2007). Humour styles, subjective well-being, trait anger, and anxiety among university students in Turkey. *World Applied Sciences Journal*, 2(5), 464-469.

Billing, A. and Moos, R. (1981). The role of coping responses and social resources in attenuating the impact of stressful life events. *Journal of Behavioural Medicine*, 4, 139-157.

Billing, A. and Moos, R. (1985). Life stressors and social resources affect post-treatment outcomes among depressed patients. *Journal of Abnormal Psychology*, 94, 140-153.

Bishop, M., Frain, M.P. and Tschopp, M.K. (2008). Self-management, perceived control and subjective quality of life in multiple sclerosis. *Rehabilitation Counselling Bulletin*, 52(1), 45-56.

Booth-Kewley, S. and Friedman, H.S. (1987). Psychological predictions of heart disease: A quantitative review. *Psychological Bulletin*, 101, 343-362.

Bower, J.E., Kemeny, M.E., Taylor, S.E., and Fahey, J.L. (1998). Cognitive processing, discovery of meaning, CD4 decline and AIDS related mortality among bereaved HIV sero positive men. *Journal of Consulting and Clinical Psychology*, 66, 979-986.

Bradburn, N.M. (1969). *The Structure of Psychological well-being.* Chicago: Aldine.

Brandtsaedter, J. and Rothermund, K. (1994). Self-percepts of control in middle and later adulthood: Buffering losses by rescaling goals. *Psychology and Aging*, 9, 265-273.

Bradley, C., Deborah, S., Gamsu Jennifer L. Moses; Graham

Knight; Andrew J.M. Boulton; John Drury; John D. Ward (1987). The use of diabetes specific perceived control and health beliefs measures to predict treatment choice and efficacy in a feasibility study of continuous subcutaneous insulin infusion pumps. *Psychology and Health*, 1476-8321, Volume 1, Issue 2, 133-146.

Braverman, S. (1983). *The relationship of social support to health*. Canadian Family Physician, 29, 559-568.

Bryant, F.B. and Veroff, J. (1982). The structure of psychological well-being: A socio-historical analysis. *Journal of Personality and Social Psychology*, 43, 653-673.

Brickman, P., Rabionowitz, V.C., Karuza, J., Coates, D., Cohn, E.M. and Kidder, L. (1982). Models of helping and coping. *American Psychologist*, 37, 368-384.

Burish, T.C. and Bradly, L.A. (1983). *Coping with Chronic Disease: Research and Application*. New Yark: Academic Press.

Calfee, C.S., Katz, P.P., Yelin, E.H., Iribarr, C., Eisner, M.D. (2006). The influencing perceived control of Asthma on health outcomes. *CHEST*, 190(5), 1812-1818.

Campbell, A., Converse, P.E. and Rodgers, W.L. (1976). *The Quality of American Life: Perception, Evaluation and Satisfaction*. New York: Russell Sage Foundation.

Canada, A.L., Parker, P.A., de moor, J.S., Basen-Engguist, K., Ramondetta, L.M. and Cohen, L. (2006). Active coping mediates the association between religion/spirituality and quality of life in Ovarian cancer. *Gynecological Oncology*, 101(1), 102-7.

Cantril, H. (1964). The Human Design. *Journal of Individual Psychology*, 20, 129-136.

Caplan, G. (1974). *Support Systems and Community Mental Health: Lectures on Concept Developments*. New York: Behavioural Publications.

Carney, R.M., Rich, M.W., TeVelde, A., Saini, J. and Jaffe, A.S. (1987). Major depressive disorders in coronary artery disease. *American Journal of Cardiology*, 60, 1273-5.

Carpenter, B.N. and Scott, S.M. (1992). Interpersonal aspects of Coping. In B.N. Carpenter (eds.) *Personal Coping: Theory, Research and Application* (pp. 93-109). New York: Praeger.

Carver, C.S. and Gaines, J. (1987). Optimism, pessimism and post-partum depression. *Cognitive Therapy and Research*, 11, 449-462.

Carver, C.S., Lehman, J.M. and Antoni, M.H. (2003). Dispositional pessimism predicts illness-related disruption of social and recreational activities among breast cancer patients. *Journal of Personality and Social Psychology*, 84, 813-821.

Carver, C.S., Pozo, C., Harris, S.D., Noriega, V., Scheier, M.F., Robinson, D.S., Ketcham, A.S., Moffat, F.L. and Clark, K.C. (1993). How coping mediates the effect of optimism on distress: A study on women with early stage breast cancer. *Journal of Personality and Social Psychology*, 65, 375-390.

Carver, C.S. and Scheier, M.F. (1981). *Attention and Self-Regulation: A Control Theory Approach to Human Behaviour*. New York: Springer-Verlag.

Carver, C.S. and Scheier, M.F. (1983). A control theory model of normal behaviour and implications for problems in self-management. In P.C. Kendall (eds.) *Advances in Cognitive behavioural research and therapy* (Vol. 2, pp. 127-194). New York: Academic Press.

Carver, C.S. and Scheier, M.F. (1985). Self-consciousness, expectancies and coping process. In T. Field, P.M. Mccabe and N. Schneiderman (eds.) *Stress and Coping* (pp. 305-330). Hillsdale, NJ: Erlbaum.

Carver, C.S. and Scheier, M.F. (1998). *On Self-Regulation of Behaviour*. New York: Cambridge University Press.

Carver, C.S., Scheier, M.F. and Pozo, C. (1992). Conceptualizing the process of coping with health problems. In H.S. Friedmen (eds.) *Hostility, Coping and Health* (pp. 167-187). Washington, DC.: American Psychological Association.

Carver, C.S., Scheier, M.F. and Weintraub, J. (1989). Assessing coping strategies: A Theoretically based approach. *Journal of Personality and Social Psychology*, 56, 267-283.

Cassileth, B.R., Lusk, E.J., Strouse, T.B., Miller, D.S., Brown, L.L., Cross, P.A. and Tenaglia, A.N. (1984). Psychosocial status in chronic illness. *The New England Journal of Medicine*, 311, 506-511.

Carvey, M.P. and Burish, T.G. (1988). Etiology and treatment of the psychological side effects associated with cancer chemotherapy: A critical review and discussion. *Psychological Bulletin*, 104, 307-325.

Cattell, R.B., Eber, H.W. and Tatsuoka, M.M. (1970). Handbook of Sixteen Personality Factor Questionnaire. Champoign II: *Institute of Personality and Ability Testing*.

Chang, E.C. (1996). Evidence of cultural specificity of pessimism in Asians vs. Caucasians: A test of a general negativity hypothesis. *Personality and Individual Differences*, 21, 819-922.

Chattopadhya, A. and A.V. Ramanakumar (2005). Burden of diseases in Rural India: An Analysis Through Cause of Death. *The Internet Journal of Third World Medicine*. Volume 2 Number 2.

Chaturvedi, A.K. (1996). Evidence for the cultural specificity of pessimism in Asians vs. Caucasians: A test of a general negativity hypothesis. *Personality and Individual Differences*, 21, 819-822.

Christensen, A.J., Turner, C.W., Smith, T.W., Holen, J.M. Jr. and Gregary, M.C. (1992). Health laws of control and depression in end stage renal disease. *Journal of Consulting and Clinical Psychology*, 59, 419-424.

Coelho, R., Amorim, I. and Prata, J. (2003). Coping styles and quality of life in patients with non-insulin dependent diabetes mellitus. *Psychosomatics*, 44, 312-318.

Cohen, S. and Lazarus, R.S. (1973). Active coping dispositions and recovery from surgery. *Psychosomatic Medicine*, 35, 375-389.

Cohen, S., Tyrell, D.A. and Smith, A.P. (1991). Psychological stress and susceptibility to the cold. *New England Journal of Medicine*, 325, 606-612.

Cohen, S. and Williconson, G.M. (1991). Stress and infectious diseases in humans. *Psychological Bulletin*, 5, 109-149.

Cohen, S. and Wills, T.A. (1985). Stress, social support and the buffering hypothesis. *Psychological Bulletin*, 98, 310-357.

Coons, S.J. and Kaplan, R.M. (1992). Assessing health related quality of life: Application to drug therapy. *Clinical Therapeutics*, 14, 850-858.

Cooper, T., Detre, T. and Weiss, S.M. (1981). Coronary prone behaviour and coronary heart disease: A critical review. *Circulation*, 63, 1199-1215.

Costa, P.T. (1987). Influence of the normal personality dimension of neuroticism on chest pain symptoms and coronary artery disease. *American Journal of Cardiology*, 60, 20-26.

Costa, P.T. and McCrae, R.R. (1985). Hypochondriasis, neuroticism and aging: When are somatic complaints unfounded? *American Psychologist*, 40, 19-28.

Costacou, T. and Mayer-Davis, E.J. (2003). Nutrition and prevention of Type II diabetes. *Annual Review of Nutrition*, 23, 147-170.

Coyne, J.C. and Delongis, A.M. (1986). Going beyond social

support: The role of social relationship in adaptation. *Journal of Consulting and Clinical Psychology*, 54, 454-460.

Coyne, J.C. and Smith, D. (1991). Couples coping with a myocardial infarction: a contextual perspective of wives' distress. *Journal of Personality and Social Psychology*, 61(3), 404-412.

Cozzarelli, C. (1993). Personality and Self-Efficacy as predictors of coping with abortion. *Journal of Personality and Social Psychology*, 65, 1224-1236.

Criqui, M.H. (1986). Epidemiology of atherosclerosis: An updated overview. *American Journal of Cardiology*, 57, 18-32.

Croog, S.H. and Levine, S. (1977). *The Heart Patient Recovers*. New York: Human Sciences Press.

Curbow, B., Somerfield, M.R., Baker, F., Wingard, J.R. and Legro, M.W. (1993). Personal changes, dispositional optimism, and psychological adjustment to bone marrow transplantation. *Journal of Behavioural Medicine*, 16, 432-466.

Cwikel, J.G., Behar, L.C., Zabora, J.R. (1997). Psychosocial factors that affect the survival of adult cancer patients: A review of research. *Journal of Psychosocial Oncology*, 15: 1-34.

Dakof, G.A. and Taylor, S.E. (1990). Victim's perception of social support: What is helpful from whom? *Journal of Personality Assessment*, 58, 80-89.

Dazord, A., Augier-Astolfi, F., Guisti, P. and Frot-Coutaz, E. (1995). Quality of life and socio-professional rehabilitation: study on patients with chronic mental diseases. *European Psychiatry*, 11(6), 277-285.

Deary, I.J. and Frier, B.M. (1995). Personality, stress and diabetes. In C.D. Spielbergor and I.G. Sarason (eds.) *Series in Stress and Emotion: Anxiety, Anger and Curiosity* (Vol. 15, pp. 33-49). Washington, DC.: Taylor and Francis.

De Boer, M.F., Ryckman, R.M., Pruyn, J.F.A. and Van den Borne, H.W. (1999). Psychosocial correlates of cancer relapse and survival: A literature review. *Patient Education Counselling*, 37: 215-230.

Deepa, R., Arvind, K. and Mohan, V. (2002). Diabetes and risk factors for coronary artery disease. *Current Science*, Vol. 83, No. 12-25, 1497-1505.

Delongis, A. and O'Brien, T. (1990). An interpersonal framework for stress and coping: An application to the families of Alzhemer's patients. In M.A.P. Stephers, J.H. Crowther, S.E.

Hobfoll and D.C. Tennenbaum (eds.) *Stress and Coping in Later Life Families*, (pp. 221-234). Washington, DC.: Hemisphere.

deRidder, D.T.D. and Schreurs, K.M.G. (1994). Coping and social support in patients with chronic disease. Report for Dutch commission for chronic diseases, Utrecht: *Section of Clinical and Health Psychology*.

Diener, E. (1994). Assessing subjective well-being: Progress and opportunities. *Social Indicators Research*, 31, 103-157.

Diener, E. and Diener, C. (1995). Most people are happy. *Psychological Science*, 7, 181-185.

Diener, E. and Emmons, R. (1984). The independence of positive and negative affect. *Journal of Personality and Social Psychology*, 47, 1105-1117.

Diener, E. and Emmons, R., Larson, R.J. and Griffin, S. (1985). The satisfaction with life scale. *Journal of Personality Assessment*, 49, 71-75.

DiMatteo, M.R. (2004). Social support and patient adherence to medical treatment: a meta-analysis. *Health Psychology*, 23, 207-218.

Dunkel-Schetter, C., Folkman, S. and Lazarus, R.S. (1987). Correlates of social support receipt. *Journal of Personality and Social Psychology*, 53, 71-80.

Dunkel-Schetter, C., Peinstein, L.G., Taylor, S.E. and Falke, R.L. (1992). Patterns of coping with cancer. *Health Psychology*, 11, 79-87.

Dura, J.R. and Beck, S.R. (1988). A comparison of family functioning when mothers have chronic pain. *Pain*, 35, 74-90.

Godfrey, J.R. (2004). Toward optimal health: The experts discuss therapeutic humour. *Journal of Women's Health*, 13, 474-479.

Eckenrode, J. (1983). The mobilization of social supports: Some individual constraints. *American Journal of Community Psychology*, 11, 509-527.

Eiser C. and Tooke, J.E. (1995). Quality of life in type II diabetes. Evaluation and applications. *Pharmacoeconomic*; 8 (Suppl 1): 17-22.

Enas, E.A. (1996). The essence and nonsense of stress: The straw that breaks the camel's back. *AAPI Journal*; 8: 47-48.

Endler, N.S. and Parker, J.D.A. (1990). Multidimensional assessment of coping: A critical evaluation. *Journal of Personality and Social Psychology*, 58, 844-854.

Endler, N.S. and Parker, J.D.A. and Summerfeldt, L.J. (1993).

Coping with health problems: Conceptual and methodological issues. *Canadian Journal of Behavioural Sciences*, 25, 384-399.

England, S.L. and Evans, J. (1992). Patients' choices and perceptions after an invitation to participate in treatment decision. *Social Science Medicine*, 34, 1217-1225.

Engle, G.L. (1977). The need for new medical models: A challenge for biomedicine. *Science*, 196, 129-136.

Epstein, S. and Meier, P. (1989). Constructive Thinking: A broad coping variable with specific components. *Journal of Personality and Social Psychology*, 57, 332-350.

Eriksen, W. (1994). The role of social support in the pathogenesis of coronary heart disease. A literature review. *Family Process*; 11: 201-09.

Eysenck, H.J. and Eysenck, M.W. (1985). *Personality and Individual Differences*. New York: Plenum.

Feather, N.T. (1982). *Expectation and actions: Expectancy value in Psychology*. Hillsdale, N.J.: Earlbaum.

Feldman, P.J., Cohen, S., Doyle, W.J., Skoner, D.P. and Gwaltney, J.M. Jr. (1999). The impact of personality on reporting of unfounded symptoms and illness. *Journal of Personality and Social Psychology*, 77(2), 370-378.

Felton, B.J., Revenson, T.A. and Hinrichson, G.A. (1984). Stress and coping in the explanation of psychological adjustment among chronically ill adults. *Social Science Medicine*, 18, 889-898.

Fingerman, K.L. and Perlmutter, M. (1995). Future time perspective and life events across adulthood. *Journal of General Psychology*, 122(1), 95-111.

Folkman, S. and Lazarus, R.R. (1980). An analysis of coping in a middle aged community sample. *Journal of Health and Social Behaviour*, 21, 219-239.

Folkman, S. and Lazarus, R.R. (1985). If it changes it must be a process: Study of emotion and coping during three stages of college examination. *Journal of Personality and Social Psychology*, 48, 150-170.

Fondacaro, M. and Moos, R. (1987). Social support and coping: A longitudinal analysis. *American Journal of Community Psychology*, 15, 653-673.

Fontana, A.F., Kerns, R.D., Rosenberg, R.L. and Colonese, K.L. (1989). Support, stress and recovery from heart disease: A Longitudinal causal model. *Health Psychology*, 8, 175-193.

Feifel, H. and Strack, S. (1989). Coping with conflict situations: Middle aged and elderly men. *Psychology and Aging*, 4(1), 26-33.

Fischer, M. and Leitchberg, H. (1986). Optimism and pessimism in elementary school aged children. *Child Development*, 57, 241-248.

Fisher, L. and Weihs, K.L. (2000) Can addressing family relationships improve outcomes in chronic disease? Report of the national working group on family-based interventions in chronic disease. *Journal of Family Practice*, 49, 561-566.

Frank, L.K. (1939). Time perspective. *Journal of Social Philosophy*, 4, 293-312.

Frans, P., Kupper, N. and Adriaasnse, M.C. (2010). Does Emotional stress cause Type 2 diabetes mellitus? A review from the European Depression In Diabetes (EDID) research consortium. *Discovery Medicine*, 9(45): 112-118.

Franks, H.M. and Roesch, S.C. (2006). Appraisals and coping in people living with cancer: A Metaanalysis. *Psycho Oncology*. 15, 1027-1037.

Franz, M.J., Bantle, J.P., Beebe, C.A., Brunzell, J.D., Chiasson, J.L., Garg, A., Holzmeister, L.A., Hoogwerf, B., Mayer-Davis, E., Mooradian, A.D., Purnell, J.Q., Wheeler, M. and American Diabetes Association. (2004) Nutrition principles and recommendations in diabetes. *Diabetes Care* 27 (Suppl 1): S36-S46.

French, R.D. (1984). The long-term relationship of marked people. In E.E. Jones, A. Farina, A.M. Hastorf, M. Marlous, D.T. Miller, and R.A. Scott (eds.) *Social Stigma: The Psychology of Marked Relationships* (pp. 255-294).

Frenzel, M.P., McCaul, K.D., Glasgero, R.E. and Schafer, L.L. (1988). The relationship of stress and coping to regimen adherence and glycemic control of diabetes. *Journal of Social and Clinical Psychology*, 6, 77-78.

Friedman, W.J. (2000). The development of children's knowledge of the times of future events. *Child Development*, 71(4), 913-32.

Friedman, M., Rosenman, R.H. (1974). *Type A behaviour and your heart*. New York: Knopf.

Furze, G. and Lewin, B. (2002). Causal attributions for angina: results of an interview study. *Coronary Health Care*, 4(3), 130-134.

Garssen, B. (2002). Psycho-oncology and cancer: Linking

psychosocial factors with cancer development. *European Society for Medical Oncology*, 171-175.

Gentry, W.D., Foster, S. and Haney, T. (1972). Denial as a determinant of anxiety and perceived health status in coronary care unit. *Psychosomatic Medicine*, 34, 39-44.

Ghulam, R., Gupta, S.R., Bandopadhyay, R.S. and Misra, S.N. (1990). Coronary prone behaviour and coronary prone disease. *Indian Journal of Psychiatry*, 32, 35-38.

Given, C.W., Stommel, M., Given, B., Osuch, J., Kurtz, M.E. and Kurtz, J.C. (1993). The influence of cancer patients symptoms and functional states on patients' depression and family caregivers' reaction and depression. *Health Psychology*, 12, 277-285.

Glass, D.C., McKnight, J.D. and Valdimarsdottir, H. (1993). Depression, burnout and perception of control in hospital nurses. *Journal of Consulting and Clinical Psychology*, 61, 147-155.

Gonder-Fredrick, L.A., Carter, W.R., Cox, D.J. and Clarke, W.L. (1990). Environmental stress and blood glucose change in insulin dependent diabetes mellitus. *Health Psychology*, 9, 503-515.

Gottlieb, B.H. (1993). Stress and coping processes in close relationships. In J. Eckenrode (eds.) *The Social Context of Stress*. New York: Plenum.

Grace, G.D. and Schill, I. (1986). Social support and coping differences in subjects high and low in interpersonal trust. *Psychological Reports*, 59, 584-586.

Grassi, L. and Molinari, S. (1986). Intrafamilial dynamics and neoplasia: Prospects for a multidisciplinary analysis. *Rivista di Psichiatria*, 21, 329-341.

Grassi, L., Biancosino B., Marmai L., Rossi E., Sabato S. (2007). Psychological Factors Affecting Oncology Conditions. In Porcelli P., Sonino N. (eds.) Psychological Factors Affecting Medical Conditions: A New Classification for DSM-V. (pp. 57-71) *Advance Psychosomatic Medicine*, Basel, Karger, Vol. 28.

Grayden, J.E. (1988). Factors that predict patients functioning following treatment for cancer. *International Journal of Nursing Studies*, 25, 117-124.

Greenwood, D.C., Muir, K.R., Packham, C.J. and Madeley, R.J. (1996). Coronary heart disease: a review of the role of psychosocial stress and social support. *Journal of Public Health Medicine*, 18: 221-31.

Grey, M., Cameron, M.E. and Thurber, F.W. (1991). Coping and adaptation in children with diabetes. *Nursing Researches*, 40, 144-149.

Griffin, K.W. and Rabkin, J.G. (1998). Perceived control over illness, realistic acceptance and psychological adjustment in people with AIDS. *Journal of Social and Clinical Psychology*, 17, 407-424.

Grob, A., Stetsenko, A., Sabatier, C., Bothjcheva, L. and Macek, P. (1999). Across national model of subjective well-being in adolescence. In F.D. Alsaker, and A. Flammer (eds.) The Adolescence Experience: European and American Adolescents in the 1990s. *Research Monograph in Adolescence* (pp. 115-130). Matiwah, N.J.: Earlbaum.

Haan, N. (1965). Coping and defense mechanism as related to personality inventories. *Journal of Consulting Psychology*, 29, 373-378.

Haidt, J. and Rodin, J. (1999). Control and efficacy as interdisciplinary bridges. *Rev. General. Psychology*. 3: 317-37.

Harkins, S.W., Price, D.D. and Braith, J. (1989). Effects of extraversion and neuroticism on experimental pain, clinical pain and illness behaviour. *Pain*, 36, 209-218.

Hanstead, B.R. (1993). Self-reported quality of life and the effect of different clinical and demographic characteristics in people with Type I diabetes. *Diabetes and Clinical Practices*, 19(2), 139-149.

Hawkley L. and Cacioppo, J. (2003). Loneliness and pathways to disease. *Brain Behaviour. Immunology*. 17: S98-105.

Heady, B. and Wearing, A. (1991). Subjective well-being: A stock and flows framework. In F. Strack, M. Argyle, and N. Schwartz (eds.) *Subjective Well-being: An interdisciplinary perspective*. USA: Pergmon Press.

Heim, E., Augusting, K., Burki, C. (1987). Coping with breast cancer: A Longitudinal prospective study. *Psychotherapy and Psychosomatic*, 48, 44-59.

Helgeson, V.S. (1992). Moderators of the relation between perceived control and adjustment to chronic illness. *Journal of Personality and Social Psychology*, 63, 656-666.

Heller, D., Watson, D. and Itlies, R. (2004). The role of person vs. situation in life satisfaction: A critical examination. *Psychological Bulletin*, 130, 574-600.

Helz, J.W. and Templeton, M.D. (1990). Evidence of the role of psychosocial factors in diabetes mellitus: A review. *American Journal of Psychiatry*, 147, 1275-1282.

Hepburn, D.A., Deary, I.J., Macleod, K.M. and Frier, B.M. (1994). Structural equation modelling of symptoms, awareness and fear of hypoglycemia and personality in patients with insulin treated diabetes. *Diabetes Care*, 17, 1273-1280.

Herpertz, S., Johann, B., Lichtblau, K., Stadtbaumer, M., Kocnar, M., Kramer-Paust, R., Heinemann, H. and Senf, W. (2000). *Patients with diabetes mellitus: Psychosocial Stress and use of psychosocial support: A Multicenter study. Med Klin (Munich)*, 15; 95(7): 369-77.

Hirsch, B. (1980). Natural support system in coping with life changes. *American Journal of Community Psychology*, 8, 159-173.

Hobfall, S.E. (1988). *The Ecology of Stress*. New York: Hemisphere.

Holahan, C.J. and Moos, R.H. (1986). Personality, coping and family resources in stress resistance: A longitudinal analysis. *Journal of Personality and Social Psychology*, 51, 389-395.

Holahan C.J and Moos R.H. (1987). Personal and contextual determinants of coping strategies. *Journal of Personality and Social Psychology*, 52, 946-955.

Homles, J.A. and Stevanson, C.A. (1990). Differential effects of avoidant and attentional coping strategies: An adaptation to chronic recent onset pain. *Health Psychology*, 9, 577-584.

Hooker, K., Monahan, D., Shiffrin, K. and Hutchison, C. (1992). Mental and physical health of spouse caregivers: The role of personality. *Psychology and Aging*, 7, 367-375.

Horquist, J.O. (1989). Quality of life: Concept and assessment. *Scandinavian Journal of Social Medicine*, 18, 69-70.

House, J.S., Kessler, R.C., Herzog, A.R., Mero, R.P., Kinney, A.M. and Breslow, M.J. (1990). Age, socio-economic status and health. *The Milbanic Quarterly*, 68, 383-411.

Hwu, Y.J. (1995). The impact of chronic illness on patients. *Rehabilitation Nursing*, 20(4), 221-5.

Ickovics, J.R. and Park, C.L. (Eds. I.) (1998). Thriving: Broadening the paradigm beyond illness to health [Special issue]. *Journal of Social Issues*, 54(2).

Indrayan, A. (2005). Forecasting vascular disease cases and associated mortality in India. Burden of Disease in India by National Commission on Macroeconomics and Health.

Iozzo P, Chareonthaitawee P., Rimoldi O., Betteridge D.J, Camici

P.G., Ferrannini E. (2002). Mismatch between insulin-mediated glucose uptake and blood flow in the heart of patients with type II diabetes. *Diabetologia,* 45: 1404-1409.

Iwanga, M., Yokoyama, H. and Seiwa, H. (2004). Coping availability and stress reduction for optimistic and pessimistic individuals. *Personality and Individual Differences,* 36(1), 11-22.

Jackuck, S.J., Brierly, H., Jackuck, S. and Wilcox, P.M. (1982). The effects of hypertensive drugs on the quality of life. *Journal of Royal College of Medical Practitioners,* 32, 103-105.

Janis, I.L. (1974). Vigilence and decision making in personal crisis. In G.V. Coelho, D.A. Hamburg and J.E. Adams (eds.) *Coping and Adaptation* (pp. 139-175). New York: Basic Books.

Janoff-Bulman, R. and McPherson Frantz, C. (1997). The impact of trauma on meaning: From meaningless world to meaningful life. In M. Power and C.R. Brewin (Eds.), *The Transformation of meaning in Psychological Therapies: Integrating Theory and Practice* (pp. 91-106). New York: Wiley.

Jeffery, R.W. (1992). Is obesity a risk factor for cardiovascular diseases? *Annals of Behavioural Medicine,* 14, 109-112.

Kahn, R.L., Wolfe, D.M., Quinn, R.P. Snock, D. and Rosenthal, R.A. (1964). *Organizational Stress: Studies in Role Conflict and Ambiguity.* New York: Wiley.

Kakar, S. (1982). *Shamans, mystics and doctors: A Psychological inquiry into India and as healing tradition.* New Delhi: Oxford University Press.

Kaplan, R.M. and Hartwell, S.L. (1987). Differential effects of social support and social network in psychological and social outcomes in men and women with Type II diabetes mellitus. *Health Psychology,* 6, 387-398.

Kaplan, R.M. and Reynolds, P. (1988). Depression and cancer mortality and morbidity: Prospective evidence from Alameda County Study. *Journal of Behavioural Medicine,* 11, 1-3.

Kapoor, N., Ahmed, H. and Ahmed, S. (1987). Psychological trait analysis of cancer patients. *Journal of Personality and Clinical Studies,* 3, 75-80.

Kaushik, S.S., Mukhopadhyay, A., Sheik, K. and Goel, S.K. (1991). A comparative study of male and female CHD patients on some psychological correlates. *Indian Journal of Clinical Psychology,* 17, 49-53.

Khare, K.C., Raman, P.G., Bhatnagar, A.D. and Bhavsar, R. (2000).

Serum Lp(a) levels in patients of diabetes mellitus. *International Journal of Diabetes in Developing Countries*, 20, 79-83.

Kidd, L., Hubbard, G., Carroll, R. and Kearney, N. (2008). Perceived control and involvement in self-care in patients with colorectal cancer. *Journal of Clinical Nursing*, 18, 2292-2300.

Kinney, T. and Coyle, K. (1989). *Predicting life satisfaction among physically disabled: Leisure's contribution*. Unpublished Report. Department of Recreation and Leisure Studies. Philadelphia Temple University.

Kjedstadli, K., Tyssen, R., Gronvold, N.T., Ekeberg, O. and Vaglum, P. (2006). Life satisfaction and resilience in medical school: A six year longitudinal nationwide and comparative study. *BMC Medical Education*, 6, 48-56.

Kleinman, A., Eisenberg, L. and Good, B. (1988). Culture, illness and care: Clinical lessons from anthropologic and cross-cultural researches. *Journal of Internal Medicine*, 88, 251-58.

Klinberg, S.L. (1967). Changes in outlook on the future between childhood and adolescence. *Journal of Personality and Social Psychology*, 7, 185-193.

Kobassa, S.C. (1979). Stressful life events, personality and health: An enquiry. *Journal of Personality and Social Psychology*, 37, 1-11.

Kobassa, S.C., Maddi, S.R. and Kahn, S. (1982). Hardiness and Health: A prospective study. *Journal of Personality and Social Psychology*, 42, 168-172.

Kothari, S. and Agarwal, M. (1999). Coping patterns among patients undergoing major surgery. *Psycho-Lingua*, 29(1), 69-76.

Krantz, D.S. and McCeney, M.K. (2002). Effects of psychological and social factors on organic disease: A critical assessment of research on coronary heart disease. *Annual Review of Psychology*, 53, 341-369.

Kubzansky, L.D., Wright, R.J., Cohen, S., Weiss, S. and Rosner B. *et al*. (2002). Breathing easy: a prospective study of optimism and pulmonary function in the normative aging study. *Annals of Behavioural Medicine*, 24: 345-53.

Kuiper, Nicholas A. and Rod A. Martin (1998). Is sense of humour a positive personality characteristic? In Ruch, W. (ed.), *The Sense of Humour: Explorations of a Personality Characteristic*. Berlin/New York: Mouton de Gruyter, 159-178.

Lang, F.R. and Cartensen, L.L. (2002). Time counts: Future time perspective, goals and social relationships. *Psychological Aging*, 17(1), 125-39.

Lazarus, R.R. (1993). Coping theory and research: Past, present and future. *Psychosomatic Medicine*, 55, 234-247.

Lazarus, R.R. and Folkman, S. (1984). *Stress Appraisal and Coping*. New York: Springer.

Lee, C.O. (1997). Quality of life and breast cancer survivors. *Psychosocial and treatment issues. Cancer Practice*, 5(5): 309-16.

Lefcourt, H.M. (1991). Locus of control. In J.P. Robinson, P.R. Shaver, and L.S. Wruightsman (eds.) *Measures of Personality and Social Psychological Attitudes* (Vol. 1, pp. 413-499). San Diego, A.: Academic Press.

Lenexa, R.D., Scott-Lenexa, J.A. and Bohlig, E.M. (1993). The cost of depression-complicated alcoholism health-care utilization and treatment effectiveness. *Journal of Mental Health Administration*; 20(Summer): 138-52.

Lennings, C.J. (2000). Optimism, satisfaction and time perspective in elderly. *International Journal of Aging and Human Development*, 51(3), 167-81.

Lepowski, Z.J. (1988). Somatization: The concept and its clinical application. *American Journal of Psychiatry*, 145, 1358-1368.

Lessing, E.E. (1985). Demographic development and personality correlates of length of future time perspective. *Journal of Personality*, 36, 183-201.

Levenson, J.L., Mishra, A., Hamer, R.M. and Hastillo, A. (1989). Denial and medical outcome in unstable angina. *Psychosomatic Medicine*, 51, 27-35.

Levine, LJ., Warrenburg, S., Kerms, R., Schwartz, G., Detaney, R., Fontana, A., Gradman, A., Smith, S., Allen, S. and Cascione, R. (1987). The role of denial in recovery from coronary heart disease. *Psychosomatic Medicine*, 49, 107-117.

Lewin, K. (1948). Time perspective and Morale. In K. Lewin (eds.) *Resolving Social Conflicts*. New York: Harper Brothers.

Lewinshon, P.M., Render, J.E. and Seely, J.R. (1991). The relationship between life satisfaction and psychosocial variables: New Perspectives. In F. Strack, Micheal Argyle and Norbert Schwartz (Eds.) *Subjective well-being: An Interdisciplinary Perspective* (pp. 143-169) England: Pergamon Press.

Litt, M.D. (1988). Self-efficacy and perceived control: Cognitive mediators. *Journal of Personality and Social Psychology*, 149-160.

Litt, M.D., Tennen, H., Affleck, G. and Klock, S. (1992). Coping and cognitive factors in adaptation to In Virto Fertilization failure. *Journal of Behavioural Medicine*, 15, 171-187.

Littlefield, C.H., Rodin, G.M., Murray, M.A. and Craven, J.L. (1990). Influence of functional impairment and social support on depressive symptoms in persons with diabetes. *Health Psychology*, 9, 737-749.

Lomranz, J., Friedman, A., Gitter, G., Shmotkin, D. and Medini, G. (1985). The meaning of time related concepts across the life span: An Israeli sample. *International Journal of Aging and Human Development*, 21(2), 87-107.

Long, B.C. and Sangster, J.L. (1993). Dispositional optimism/ pessimism and adjustment of rheumatoid and osteoarthritis patients. *Journal of Applied Social Psychology*, 23, 1069-1091.

Luscombe, F.A. (2003). Health related quality of life and associated psychosocial factors in irritable bowel syndrome: A Review. *Journal of Urology*, 169(1), 233-6.

Lynch, J.J. (1977). *The Broken heart: The medical consequences of loneliness*. New York: Basic Books.

Lyons, R. (1986). *The impact of chronic illness on activity patterns and friendships* (Research Report). Ottawa: Fitness and Life Style Research Institute.

Lyons, R. (1991). *The effects of acquired illness and disability on friendships* (Vol. 3, pp. 223-277). London: J. Kingslay.

Macintyre, S. and Pritchard, C. (1989). Comparisons between self-assessed and observer assessed presence and severity of colds. *Social Science Medicine*, 29, 1243-1248.

Maes, S. and Bruggemans, F. (1990). Approach-avoidance and illness behaviour in coronary heart patients. In L.R. Schmidt, P. Schwenknezger, J. Weinman and S. Maes (eds.) *Theoretical and Applied Aspects of Health Psychology* (pp. 297-308). Chur, Switzerland: Harwood.

Manne, S. and Zautra, A.J. (1989). Spouse criticism and support: Their association with coping and psychological adjustment among women with rheumatoid arthritis. *Journal of Personality and Social Psychology*, 56(4), 608-617.

Manne, S.L., Ostroff, J., Winkel G., Fox K., and Grana G. (2005a). Partner unsupportive responses, avoidant coping, and distress among women with early stage breast cancer: patient and partner perspectives. *Health Psychology*, 24: 635-41.

Manning-Walsh, J. (2005). Social support as a mediator between symptom distress and quality of life in women with breast cancer. *Journal of Obstetric Gynecology Neonatal Nursing*, July-Aug. 34(4): 482-93.

Marcowitz, J.H., Metthews, K.A., Wing, R.R., Kuller, L.H. and Meilahn, E.N. (1991). Psychological, biological and health behaviour predictors of blood pressure changes in middle aged women. *Journal of Hypertension*, 9, 399-406.

Martin, P. (1989). Personality and coping in survivors of myocardial infraction. *Journal of Social Behaviour and Personality*, 4, 587-601.

Maasoumeh Rambod and Forough Rafii (2010). Perceived Social Support and Quality of Life in Iranian Hemodialysis Patients. *Journal of Nursing Scholarship*, 42(3), 242-249.

Matheny, K.B., Roque-Tovar, B.E. and Curlette, W.L. (2008). Perceived stress, coping resources and life satisfaction among U.S. and Mexican college students: A cross-cultural study. *Anales de Psicologia*, 24, 49-57.

Matthews, K.A., Raikkonen K., Sutton-Tyrell K. and Kuller L.H. (2004). Optimistic attitudes protect against progression of carotid atherosclerosis in healthy middle-aged women. *Psychosomatic Medicine*, 66, 640-44.

Maunsell, E. Brisson, J., Deschenes, L. (1995). Social support and survival among women with breast cancer. *Cancer*, 76: 631-637.

Mayou, R. and Bryant, B. (1987). Quality of life after coronary artery surgery. *Quarterly Journal of Medicine*, 23, 239-248.

McCrae, R.R. (1992). *Situational determinants of Coping*. In B.N. Carpenter (eds.) Personal Coping: Theory, Research and Application (pp. 65-76). West Port, C.T.: Praeger.

McCrae, R.R. and Costa, P.T., Jr. (1984). *Emerging lives, enduring dispositions: Personality in adulthood.* Boston: Little Brown.

McCrae, R.R. and Costa P.T., Jr. (1986). Personality, coping and coping effectiveness in an adult sample. *Journal of Personality*, 54, 385-405.

Meade, R.D. (1972). Future time perspectives of Americans and sub-cultures in India. *Journal of Cross-Cultural Psychology*, Vol. 3, No. 1, 93-99.

Miller, S.M. (1979). Controllability and Human Stress: Method, evidence and theory. *Behaviour Research and Theory*, 17, 287-306.

Mishra, M. and Agarwal, A. (2003). Coping and satisfaction with life in working women. In A. Agarwal and A.K. Saxena (eds.) *Psychological Perspectives in Environmental and Developmental Issues*. New Delhi: Concept Publishing Company Pvt. Ltd.

Moos, R.H., Brenman, P.L., Fondacaro, M. and Moos, B.S. (1990).

Approach and avoidance coping responses among older problem and non-problem drinkers. *Psychology and Aging*, 5, 31-40.

Moos, R.H. and Schaefer, J.A. (1993). Coping resources and processes: Current concepts and measures. In L. Goldberger and S. Breznitz (eds.) *Handbook of Stress: Theoretical and Clinical Aspects* (end ed., pp. 234-257). New York: Free Press.

Moos, R.H. and Tsu, V.D. (1977). The crisis of physical illness. In R.H. Moos (eds.) *Coping with Physical Illness* (pp. 3-21). New York: Plenum.

Mumma, C. and McCorkle, R. (1983). Causal attribution and life threatening disease. *International Journal of Psychiatry Medicine*, 12(4), 311-9.

Murphy, D.J., Williamson, P.S. and Nease, D.E., Jr. (1994). Supportive family members of diabetic adults. *Family Practice Research Journal*, 14(4), 323-31.

Murrell, A. and Mingrone, M. (1994). Correlates of temporal perspectives. *Perceptual Motor Skills*, 78(3), 1331-4.

Myers, D. and Diener, A. (1995). *Who is happy? Psychological Science*. 6(1), 10-20.

National Cancer Registry Programme (2002). Two years report of the Population-based Cancer Registries 1997-1998. *Incidence and Distribution of Cancer*. New Delhi: Indian Council of Medical Research.

Nemeroff, C.B., Musselman, D.L. and Evans, D.L. (1998). Depression and cardiac disease. *Depress Anxiety*; 8 (suppl 1): 71-9.

Norem, J. and Cantor, N. (1996). Anticipatory and positive cushioning strategies: Optimism and defensive pessimism in 'risky' situations. *Cognitive Therapy and Research*, 10, 347-362.

Nuttin, J. (1964). Future time perspective in human motivation and learning. *Acta Psychologia*, 23, 60-82.

O'Brien, M.T. (1983). Multiple sclerosis: The relationship among self-esteem, social support and coping behaviour. *Applied Nursing Research*, 6(2), 54-63.

Ohtake T, Yokoyama I., Watanabe T., Momose T., Serezawa T., Nishikawa J., Sasaki Y. (1995). Myocardial glucose metabolism in non-insulin-dependent diabetes mellitus patients evaluated by zDG-PET. *Journal of Nuclear Medicine*, 36: 456-463.

Okosum, I.S., Liao, Y., Rotimi, C.N.M., Dever, G.E. and Cooper, R.S. (2001). Impact of birth weight on ethnic variations in subcutaneous and central adiposity in American children aged 5-11 years: A Study from third National Health and Nutrition Examination Survey. *International Journal of Obesity*, 24, 479-484.

Okum, M.A., Stock, W.A., Haring, M.J. and Witter, R.A. (1984). Health and subjective well-being: A meta analysis. *Journal of Aging and Human Development*, 19, 111-132.

O'Malley, P.G., Jones, D.L., Feuerstein, I.M. and Taylor, A.J. (2000). Lack of a correlation between psychological factors and subclinical coronary artery disease. *New England Journal of Medicine*, 343: 1298-304.

Parashar, R.P. (2000). Lifestyle for perfect health. *Psychological Studies*, 45(3), 167-172.

Park, C.L., Moore, P.J., Turner, R.A. and Adlor, N.E. (1997). The role of constructive thinking and optimism in psychological and behavioural adjustment during pregnancy. *Journal of Personality and Social Psychology*, 73, 584-592.

Parker, J.D.A. and Endler, N.S. (1992). Coping with coping assessment: A critical review. *European Journal of Psychology*, 6, 321-344.

Parkes, K.R. (1986). Coping in stressful episodes: The role of individual differences, environmental factors and situational characteristics. *Journal of Personality and Social Psychology*, 51, 1277-1292.

Patten, S.B. (1994). Long-term medical conditions and major depression conditions in the Canadian population. *Canadian Journal of Psychiatry*, 4: 151-7.

Patrick, D.L., Margan, M. and Charlton, J.R.H. (1986). Psychosocial support and change in the health status of physically disabled people. *Social Science Medicine*, 22, 1347-1354.

Pavot, W., Diener, E. and Suh, E. (1998). The Temporal Satisfaction with Life Scale. *Journal of Personality Assessment*, 70, 340-354.

Peale, N.V. (1956). *The Power of Positive Thinking*. Englewood Cliffs, N.J.: Prentice Hall.

Pennebeker, J. (1982). *The Psychology of Physical Symptoms*. New York: Springer-Verlag.

Peralin, L.I. and Schooler, C. (1978). The structure of coping. *Journal of Health and Social Behaviour*, 19, 2-21.

Peterson, C. (2000) 'Rural health and families: E-health solutions to health inequities', *Journal of Family Studies* 6(2): 298-301.

Peterson, C., Seligman, M.E.P. and Valliant, G.E. (1988). Pessimistic explanatory style is a risk factor for physical illness: A thirty years longitudinal study. *Journal of Personality and Social Psychology*, 55, 23-27.

Peterson, C. and Stunkard, A.J. (1989). Personal control and health promotion. *Social Science Medicine*, 28, 819-828.

Petticrew, M., Fraser, J.M. and Regan, M.F. (1999). Adverse life-events and risk of breast cancer: a meta-analysis. *British Journal of Health Psychology*, 4: 1-17.

Pollock, S.E. (1989). Adaptive responses to diabetes mellitus. *Western Journal of Nursing Research*, 11, 265-280.

Pouwer, F., Beekman, A.T., Nijpels, G., Dekker, J.M., Snoek, F.J., Kostense, P.J., Heine, R.J., Deeg, D.J. (2003). Rates and risks for co-morbid depression in patients with Type 2 diabetes mellitus: results from a community-based study. *Diabetologia*, 46(7): 892-898.

Praming, S., Thorsteinsson, B., Theilgard, A., Pinner, E.M. and Binder, C. (1986). Cognitive function during hypoglycemia in Type I diabetes mellitus. *British Medical Journal*, 292, 647-50.

Primeau, F. (1998). Post stroke depression: A critical review of the literature. *Canadian Journal of Psychiatry*, 33, 757-765.

Pucheu, S., Consoli, S.M., D'Auzac, C., Francais, P. and Issad, B. (2004). Do health causal attributions and coping strategies act as moderators of quality of life in peritoneal dialysis patients? *Journal of Psychosomatic Medicine*, 56(3), 317-322.

Rakowski, W. (1979). Future time perspective in later adulthood: Review and Research directions. *Experimental Aging Research*, 5(1), 43-88.

Raleigh, E.D. (1992). Sources of Hope in Chronic Illness. *Oncology Nursing Forum*, 19(3), 493-8.

Reddy, K.S. and Yusuf, S. (1998). Emerging epidemic of cardiovascular disease in developing countries. *Circulation*, 97, 596-601.

Reed, G.M., Taylor, S.E. and Kemeny, M.E. (1993). Perceived control and psychological adjustment in gay men with AIDS. *Journal of Applied Social Psychology*, 23, 791-824.

Reed, G.M., Kemeny, M.E., Taylor, S.E., Wang, H.Y.J. and Visscher, B.R. (1994). Realistic acceptance as predictor of decreased survival time in gay men with AIDS. *Health Psychology*, 13, 299-307.

Reker, G.T. and Wong, P.T.P. (1985). Personal optimism, physical and mental health: The triumph of successful aging. In J.E. Biren and J. Livingstom (eds.) *Cognition, Stress and Aging* (pp. 134-177). Englewood Cliffs, N.J.: Prentice Hall.

Renneker, R. (1981). Cancer and psychotherapy. In J.G. Goldberg (eds.) *Psychotherapeutic Treatment of Cancer Patients* (pp. 131-166). New York: Free Press.

Renneker, R. and Cutler, M. (1952). Psychological problems of the breast cancer. *Journal of American Medical Association*, 148, 833-838.

Rizvi, S.N.H. (1990). Folk concept of health and disease: A case study. *The Eastern Anthropologist*, 44, 179-188.

Rodin, J. (1986). Aging and health: Effects of the sense of control. *Science*, 233, 1271-1276.

Rodin, G. and Vorshart, K. (1986). Depression in the medically ill: An Overview. *American Journal of Psychiatry*, 143, 696-705.

Roeckelein, J.E. (2002). *The psychology of humour: A reference guide to annotated bibliography*. Westport, CT; Greenwood Press.

Rothbaum, F., Weisz, J.R., Snyder, S.S. (1982). Changing the world and changing the self. *Journal of Personality and Social Psychology*, 42, 5-27.

Rothrock, N.E., Lutegendort, S.K. and Kreder, K.J. (2003). Coping strategies in patients with interstitial cystitis: Relationship with quality of life and depression. *Diabetic Medicine*, 20(2), 135-146.

Rothspan, S. and Reed, S.J. (1996). Present *versus* future time perspective and HIV risk among heterosexual college students. *Health Psychology*, 15(2), 131-4.

Rotton, J. and Shats, M. (1998). Effects of state humour expectation and hope on post-surgical mood and self-medication: A Field experiment. *Journal of Applied Social Psychology*, 26, 1775-1794.

Salovery, P., O'Leary, A., Stretton, M.S., Fishkin, S.A. and Drake, C.A. (1991). Influence of mood on judgment about health and control. In J.P. Firgas (eds.) *Emotion and Social Developments* (pp. 241-261). New York: Pergamon Press.

Sammarco, A. and Konecny, L.M. (2008). Quality of life, social support and uncertainty among Latina Breast cancer survivors. *Oncology Nursing Forum*, 35(5), 844-9.

Santos, P.R. (2010). Correlation between coping style and quality of life among hemodialysis patients from a low income area in Brazil. *Hemodialysis International*, 14(3), 316-321.

Savli, H. and Sevinc, A. (2005). The evaluation of the Turkish version of the well-being questionnaire (WBO-22) in patients with type 2 diabetes: The effects of diabetic complications. *Journal of Endocrinology Investigation*, 28, 683-691.

Saxena, S. Chandirmani, K. and Bhargava, R. (1998). WHOQOL-Hindi: A questionnaire for assessing quality of life in health care settings in India. World Health Questionnaire Quality of Life. *National Medical Journal of India*, 11(4), 160-5.

Sastry, J. and Ross, C.E. (1998). Asian ethnicity as the sense of personal control. *Social Psychology Quarterly*, 61(2), 101-120.

Schaefer, J.A. and Moos, R.H. (1992). Life Crises and Personal Growth. In B.N. Carpenter (Ed.), *Personal coping theory, research, and application* (pp. 149-170). Westport, CT: Praeger.

Scheier, M.F. and Carver, C.S. (1985). Optimism, coping and health: Assessment and implications of generalized outcome expectancies. *Health Psychology*, 4, 219-247.

Scheier, M.F. and Carver, C.S. (1987). Dispositional optimism and physical well-being: The influence of generalized outcome expectancies on health. *Journal of Personality*, 55, 169-210.

Scheier, M.F. and Carver, C.S. (2001). Adapting to cancer: the importance of hope and purpose. In A. Baum and B.C. Anderson (eds.) *Psychosocial Intervention for Cancer* (pp. 15-36) Washington, DC.: American Psychological Association.

Scheier, M.F., Mattews, K.A., Owens, J.F., Magovern, G.J., Lefebevre, R.C., Abbott, R.A. and Carver, C.S. (1989). Dispositional optimism and recovery from coronary artery bypass surgery: The beneficial effects on physical and psychological well-being. *Journal of Personality and Social Psychology*, 57, 1024-1040.

Schultz, R., Heckhausen, J. and O'Brian, A.T. (1994). Control and disablement process in the elderly. *Journal of Social Behaviour and Personality*, 9, 139-152.

Schwartz, G.E. (1982). Testing the biopsychosocial model: The ultimate challenge facing behavioural medicine? *Journal of Consulting and Clinical Psychology*, 50, 1040-1053.

Seeman, M. and Lewis, S. (1995). Powerlessness, health, and mortality: a longitudinal study of older men and mature women. *Social Science Medicine*, 41: 517-25.

Seligman, M.E.P. (1975). *Helplessness: On Depression Development and Death*. San Francisco: Freeman.

Schram, M.T., Baan, C.A. and Pouwer, F. (2009). Depression and quality of life in patients with diabetes: a systematic review from the European Depression In Diabetes (EDID) research consortium. *Current Diabetes Review,* 5(2): 112-119.

Schwarzer, R. and Leppin, A. (1991). Social support and health: a theoretical and empirical overview. *Journal of Social and Personal Relations,* 8: 99-127.

Shaw, R.E., Cohen, F., Doyle, B. and Palesky, J. (1986). The impact of denial and aggressive style on information gain and rehabilitation outcomes in myocardial infraction patients. *Psychosomatic Medicine,* 47, 262-273.

Shell, D.F. 7 Husman, J. (2001). Time perspective beliefs in achievement and self-regulation. *Contemporary Educational Psychology,* 26(4), 481-506.

Sherbourne, C.D., Hays, R.D., Ordway, L., DiMattes, M.R. and Kravits, R.L. (1992). Antecedents of adherence to medical recommendations: Results from the medical outcomes study. *Journal of Behavioural Medicine,* 15(5), 447-468.

Shin, D.C. and Johnson, D.M. (1978). Avowed happiness as an overall assessment of the quality of life. *Social Indicators Research,* 5, 475-492.

Shiffren, K. and Hooker, K. (1995). Stability and change in optimism: A study among spouse caregivers. *Experimental Aging Research,* 21, 59-76.

Shmotkin, D. (1991). The role of time orientation in life satisfaction across the life-span. *Journal of Gerontology: Psychological Sciences,* 46, pp. 243-250.

Siegman, A.W., Anderson, R., Herbst, J., Boyle, S. and Wilkinson, J. (1992). Dimensions of anger-hostility and cardiovascular reactivity in provoked and angered men. *Journal of Behavioural Medicine,* 15, 257-272.

Silver, R.L. and Wortman, C.B. (1980). Coping with undesirable life events. In J. Garber and M.E.P. Seligman (eds.) *Human Helplessness: Theory and Applications.* New York: Academic Press.

Singh, S.B. and Misra, (1987). Stressful life events and myocardial infraction. *Indian Journal of Clinical Psychology,* 14, 77-79.

Singh, T., Misra, G. and Verma, S. (1999). Concept of health and illness in four systems of medicine: Some policy implications. In G. Misra (eds.) *Psychological perspectives on health and Stress,* New Delhi: Concept Publishing Company Pvt. Ltd.

Sinha, D. (1990). Concept of psychosocial well-being: Western and Indian perspectives. *NIMHANS Journal,* 8, 1-11.

Sinha, J.B.P. (1985). Concept of health and healing in India. *Dyamische Psychiatric*, 18, 30-42.

Skelton, M. and Pennebaker, J. (1978). Dispositional determinants of symptoms reporting: Correlational evidence. Paper presented at the annual meeting of the *American Psychological Association*. Toronto, Canada.

Smith, T.W. (1992). Hostility and Health: Current status of a psychosomatic hypothesis. *Health Psychology*, 11, 139-150.

Smith, T.W., Pope, M.K., Rhodewalt, F. and Poulton, J. (1989). Optimism, neuroticism, coping and symptoms reports: An alternative interpretation of the Life Orientation Test. *Journal of Personality and Social Psychology*, 56, 640-648.

Snyder, C.R. (1994). Hope and Optimism. In V.S. Ramchandran (eds.) *Encyclopedia of Human Behaviour* (Vol. 2, pp. 535-542). San Diego, C.A.: Academic Press.

Snyder, C., Harris, C., Anderson, J., Holleran, S., Irving, L., Sigmon, S. *et al.*, (1991). The will and the ways: Development and validation of an individual difference measure of hope. *Journal of Personality and Social Psychology*, 60, 570-585.

Solvic, P., Fischhoff, B. and Lichtenstein, S. (1977). Behavioural decision theory. *Annual Review of Psychology*, 58, 7-14.

Sowers, J.R and Epstein, M. (1995) Diabetes mellitus and associated hypertension, vascular disease, and nephropathy: An update. *Hypertension*, 26(6 Pt 1), 869-879.

Spilker, B. (1990). *Quality of Life Assessments in Clinical Trials*. New York: Raven Press.

Spirito, A., Ruggiero, L., Bower, A. and McGarvey, S.T. (1991). Stress coping and social support as mediators of emotional status of women with gestational diabetes. *Psychology and Health*, 5, 111-120.

Sridhar, G.R. and Madhu, K. (2001). Stress in the cause and course of diabetes. *International Journal of Diabetes in Developing Countries*, 21, 112-120.

Stanton, A.L. and Snider, P.R. (1993). Coping with breast cancer diagnosis: A prospective study. *Health Psychology*, 12, 16-23.

Stephens, M.A.P., Crowther, J.H., Hobfoll, S.E. and Tennenbaum, D.L. (1990). *Stress and Coping in Later Life Families*. New York: Hemisphere.

Steptoe, A. (1989). The significance of personal control in health and disease. In A. Steptoe and Aappels (eds.) *Stress, Personal Control and Health* (pp. 309-318). Brussels, Beligium: John Wiley and Sons.

Stemack, R.M. (1990). Biological bases of extraversion: Psycho physiological evidences. *Journal of Personality*, 58, 293-311.

Stillerman, L. (2006). *Humour in Relation to Anxiety, Depression and Stress for College Students*. Unpublished doctoral dissertation. New Mexico State University, Las Cruces, NM.

Strcak, S., Schwartz, N. and Gschneidhinger, E. (1985). Happiness and reminiscing: The role of time perspective affect and mode of thinking. *Journal of Personality and Social Psychology*, 49(6), 1460-1469.

Strickland, B.R. (1978). Internal-external expectancies and health related behaviours. *Journal of Consulting and Clinical Psychology*, 46, 119-121.

Suh, E.M. and Diener, E. (1999). *The use of emotion information across cultures, individuals and persons: The case of life satisfaction*. Manuscript submitted for publication. University of Illinois, Urbana-Champaign.

Suh, E.M., Diener, E. and Fujita, F. (1996). Events and subjective well-being: Only recent events matter. *Journal of Personality and Social Psychology*, 70, 1091-1102.

Sullivan, M., Edgley, K. and Dehoux, E. (1990). A survey of multiple sclerosis. Part 1: Perceived cognitive and compensatory strategy use. *Canadian Journal of Rehabilitation*, 4(2), 99-108.

Sweetman, M.E., Munz, D.C. and Wheeler, R. (1993). Optimism, hardiness and explanatory style as predictors of general well-being among attorneys. *Social Indicators Research*, 29, 153-161.

Takela, F. (1989). Quality of Life in cancer patients. *Neurosurgery Clinics*, 16, 52-58.

Taylor, S.E. (1990). Health Psychology: The Science and the Field. *American Psychology*, 45, 40-50.

Taylor, S.E. and Aspinwell, L.G. (1990). Psychological aspects of chronic illness. In G.R. VandenBos and P.T. Coasta, Jr. (eds.) *Psychological Aspects of Serious illness*. Washington, DC.: American Psychological Association.

Taylor, S.E. and Brown, J.D. (1994). Positive illusions and well-being revisited: Separating fact from fiction. *Psychological Bulletin*, 116, 21-27.

Taylor, S.E., Frier, B.M., Gold, A.E. and Deary, I.J. (2002).

Psychological factors and diabetes related outcomes following diagnosis of Type II diabetes in adults: The Edisburgh Prospective Diabetes Study. *Diabetes Care*, 25, 1154-1158.

Taylor, S.E., Helgeson, V.S., Reed, G.M. and Skokan, L.A. (1991). Self-generated feelings of control and adjustment to physical illness. *Journal of Social Issues*, 47, 91-109.

Taylor, S.E., Kemeny, M.E., Reed, G.M. and Aspinwell, L.G., (1991). Assault on the Self: Positive illusions and adjustment. In G.A. Goethals and J.A. Strauss (eds.) *The Self: An Interdisciplinary Perspective* (pp. 239-254). New York: Springer-Verlag.

Taylor, S.E., Kemeny, M.E., Aspinwell, L.G., Schneider, S.C., Rodrigwez, R. and Herbert, M. (1992). Optimism, coping, psychological distress and high risk sexual behaviour among men at risk for AIDS. *Journal of Personality and Social Psychology*, 63, 460-473.

Taylor, S.E, Lerner, J.S, Sherman, D.K, Sage, R.M, McDowell, N.K. (2003a). Portrait of the self-enhancer: well-adjusted and well-liked or maladjusted and friendless? *Journal of. Personality and Social Psychology*, 84: 165-76.

Taylor, S.E, Lerner, J.S, Sherman, D.K, Sage, R.M, McDowell, N.K. (2003b). Are self-enhancing cognitions associated with healthy or unhealthy biological profiles? *Journal of Personality and Social Psychology*, 85: 605-15.

Taylor, S.E., Lichtman, R.R. and Wood, J.V. (1984). Attributions, beliefs about control, and adjustment to breast cancer. *Journal of Personality and Social Psychology*, 46, 489-502.

Taylor, S.E. and Rochman, S.J. (1988). The effects of blood sugar changes on cognitive function, affective state and somatic symptoms. *Journal of Behavioural Medicine*, 11, 279-292.

Tedeschi, R. G., Park, C.L. and Calhoun, L.G. (Eds.). (1998). *Post-traumatic Growth: Positive Changes in the Aftermath of Crisis*. Mahwah, NJ: Erlbaum.

Temoshok, L. (1987). Personality, coping style, emotion and cancer: Towards an integrative model. *Cancer Surveys*, 6, 545-567.

Tennen, H., Affleck, G., Urrows, S., Higgins, P. and Mendola, R. (1992). Perceiving control, construing benefits and daily process in rheumatoid arthritis. *Canadian Journal of Behavioural Sciences*, 24, 186-203.

Thoits, P.A. (1986). Social support as coping assistance. *Journal of Consulting and Clinical Psychology*, 54, 416-423.

Thomas, C.B. and Duszynski, K.R. (1974). Closeness to parents and the family constellation is a prospective study of eve disease status: Suicide, mental illness, malignant tumou, hypertension and coronary heart disease. *John Hopkins Medical Journal*, 134, 251-270.

Thompson, S.C., Nanni, C. and Levine, A. (1994). Primary *versus* secondary and disease *versus* consequence related control in HIV positive men. *Journal of Personality and Social Psychology*, 67, 540-547.

Thompson, S.C., Sobolen, Shubin, A., Galbraith, M.E., Schwankovsky, L. and Cruzen, D. (1993). Maintaining perceptions of control: Finding perceived control in low control circumstances. *Journal of Personality and Social Psychology*, 64, 293-304.

Thopmson, S.C. and Wierson, M. (2000). Enhancing perceived control in psychotherapy. In C.R. Snyder and R.E. Ingram (eds.) *Handbook of Psychological Change* (pp. 177-197). New York: Wiley.

Tiger, L. (1979). *Optimism: The Biology of the Hope*. New York: Simon and Schustor.

Timmer, E., Steverink, N., Stevens, N. and Dittmann-Hohli, F. (2003). Personal concepts of stability in the second half of life. *Journal of Aging Studies*, 17, 427-443.

Tiwari, S. and Agarwal, A. (1989). Arousal of future orientation and attitude formation. *Indian Psychologists*, 6(1 and 2), 21-29.

Tobin, D.L., Holroyd, K.A., Reynolds, R.V., *et al.* (1989).: The hierarchical factor structure of the Coping Strategies Inventory. *Cognitive Therapy Research*, 13: 343-361.

Trew, M. and Maguire, P. (1982). Future comparison of two instruments for measuring quality of life in cancer patients. In J. Bedeman (eds.) *Quality of Life, Workshop of the EDRTC study Group on Quality of Life*: Paris.

Trief, P.M., Grant, W., Elbert, K and Weinstock, R.S. (1998). Family environment, glycemic control and the psychosocial adaptation of adults with diabetes. *Diabetes Care*; 21: 241-5.

Tripathi, R. (1993). *Psychosocial Factors in Health Behaviour*. Doctoral Dissertation, Department of Psychology, Allahabad University, Allahabad.

Trommsddroff, G. (1978). *Social Conditions of Future Orientation*. EASP Weimear, April.

Turk, D.C., Rudy, T.E. and Flor, H. (1986). Why a family perspective on pain? *International Journal of Family Therapy*, 7, 223-234.

Turner, J.A. and Clancy, S. (1986). Strategies for coping with low back pain: Relationship to pain and disability. *Pain*, 24, 355-364.

Upadhyay, S. (2002). *Influence of Optimism, Future Orientation and Detachment on Health in Derivational Environment*. Unpublished doctoral dissertation, Department of Psychology, D.D.U. Gorakhpur University, Gorakhpur.

Uppaluri, C.R. (2002). Heart disease and its relative risk factors in Asian Indians. *Ethnic Disease*; 12: 45-53.11, 35-42.

Vaidya, A.K., Srivastava, S.N. and Srivastava, K.B. (1985). Neuroticism in hypertensive and cancer patients. *Perspectives in Psychological Researches*, 8, 34-37.

Van Beek, W., Kerkhof, Ad. and Beekman, A. (2009). Future oriented group training for suicidal patients: A randomized clinical trial. *BMC Psychiatry*, 9, 65-79.

Veenhoven, R. (1984). *Conditions of Happiness*. Hingham, M.A.: Kluwer Boston: Academic Publisher.

Verma, S.K., Wig, N.N. and Pershad, D. (1985). *Manual for PGI Health Questionnaire N-1. Agra*: National Psychological Corporation.

Vinokur, A.D., Schul, Y. and Caplan, R.D. (1987). Determinants of perceived social support: International transactions, personal outlook and transient affect states. *Journal of Personality and Social Psychology*, 53, 1137-1145.

Voipio-Pulkki, L.M., Nuutila, P., Knuuti, M.J., Ruotsalainen, U., Haaparanta, M., Teräs, M., Wegelius, U. and Koivisto, V.A. (1993). Heart and skeletal muscle glucose disposal in type 2 diabetic patients as determined by positron emission tomography. *Journal of Nuclear Medicine*. 34(12): 2064-2067.

Von Dras, D.D. and Lichty, W. (1990). Correlates of depression in diabetic adults. *Health and Dying*, 1, 79-84.

Vosvick, M., Krumboltz, J. and Spiegel, D. (2003). Relationship of functional quality of life to strategies for coping with the stress of living with HIV/AIDS. *Psychosomatics*, 44, 51-58.

Wagner, M.K., Armstrong, D. and Laughlin (1995). Cognitive determinants of quality of life after onset cancer. *Psychological Reports*, 77, 147-154.

Wales, J.K. (1995). Does psychological stress causes diabetes? *Diabetic Medicine*, 12(2), 109-12.

Walker, K.N., MacBridge, A. and Vachon, M.L. (1977). Social support networks in the crisis of bereavement. *Social Science Medicine*, 11, 35-42.

Warr, P.B. (1978). A study of psychological well-being. *British Journal of Psychology*, 69, 111-121.

Warr, P.B. (1987). *Work, Employment and Mental Health*. Oxford: Clarendon Press.

Watson, D. and Pennebaker, J.W. (1989). Health complaints, stress and distress: Exploring the central role of negative affectivity. *Psychological Review*, 96, 234-254.

Watson, D. and Tellegon, A. (1984). Towards a consensual structure of mood. *Psychological Bulletin*, 98, 219-235.

Wearden, A.J., Hynd, K., Smith, H., Davis, R. and Tarrier, N. (2006). Idiosyncratic Personal Explanations for Blood Glucose Events are Associated with Poorer Self-Management and Glycemic Control in Adult Patients with Long-Standing Type 1 Diabetes. *Diabetes Care*, 29: 1208-1213.

Weaver, A.J. and Flannelly, K.J. (2004). The role of religion/spirituality for cancer patients and their caregivers. *South Medical Journal*, 97 (12), 1210-4.

Weinberg, N. and Williams, J. (1978). How the physically disabled perceive their disabilities. *Journal of Rehabilitation*, 44, 31-33.

Weiner, B. (1985). Spontaneous causal thinking. *Psychological Bulletin*, 97: 74-84.

Weisman, A.D. and Worden, J.W. (1976). The existential plight in cancer: Significance of the first 100 days. *International Journal of Psychiatry and Medicine*, 7, 1-15.

Wenseueir, M. and Grossman, K.E. (1998). Principles of attachment theory in subjective life satisfaction and individual orientation to the future in advanced adulthood. *Z. Gerontol Geriatr*, 31(5), 362-70.

White, N.E., Richter, J.M. and Fry, C. (1992). Coping, social support and adaptation to chronic illness. *Western Journal of Nursing Research*, 14(2), 211-224.

WHO (1947). *Constitution of the World Health Organization*, Chronicles of the World Health Organization, Switzerland: Geneva.

WHO (2002). The World Health Report 2002—Reducing risks, promoting healthy life. *World Health Organization*, Geneva, Switzerland *http://www.who.int/whr/2002/en/*

Wiebe, D.J. and Smith, T.H. (1997). Personality and health: Progress in problems in psychosomatic. In R. Hogan, J. Johnson and K.S. Brigs (eds.) *Handbook of Personality Psychology* (pp. 892-908), New York: Academic Press.

Williams, J.E., Paton, C.C., Seigler, I.C., Eigenbrodt, M.L., Nieto, F.J. and Tyroler, H.A. (2000). Anger proneness predicts coronary heart disease: Prospective analysis from the Atherosclerosis Risk In Communities (ARIC) study. *Circulation*, 101(17), 2038-9.

Wills, T.A., Sandy, JM. and Yaeger, A.M., (2001). Time perspective and early onset substance use: A model based on stress-coping theory. *Psychology of Addictive Behaviour*, 15(2), 118-25.

Wing, R.R., Goldstein, M.G., Acton, K.J., Birch, L.L., Jakicic, J.M., Sallis, J.F. Jr., Smith-West, D., Jeffery, R.W. and Surwit, R.S. (2001). Lifestyle changes related to obesity, eating behaviour and physical activity. *Diabetes Care*, 24: 117-123.

Woller, W., Kruse, J., Albert, L., Kraut, D., Riohter, B., Worth, H. and Tress, W., (1992). Coping with attacks and illness behaviour in patients with bronchial asthma. *Psychotherapie Psychosomatik urd Medizinische Psychologic*, 42, 63-70.

Wonghongkul, T. Dechaprom, N., Phumivichuvate, L. and Losawatkul, S. (2006). Uncertanity appraisal coping and quality of life in breast cancer survivors. *Cancer Nursing*, 29(3), 250-7.

Woodruff, S.L. and Convey, T.L. (1990). Perceived quality of life and health related correlates among men aboard Navy ships. *Military Psychology*, 2, 79-94.

Yokoyama, I., Yonekura, K., Ohtake, T., Kawamura, H., Matsumoto, A., Inoue, Y., Aoyagi, T., Sugiura, S., Omata, M., Ohtomo, K., Nagai, R. (2000). Role of insulin resistance in heart and skeletal muscle F-18 fluorodeoxyglucose uptake in patients with non-insulin-dependent diabetes mellitus. *Journal of Nuclear Cardiology*, 7: 242-248.

Zikmud, V., Cogan, S. and Jurkoviciva, O. (1983). Ability to cope with difficult situation in premorbid life and survival after the first myocardial infraction control after 10 years. *tivitas Norvosa Superior*, 25, 210-21.

Index